PREPARE
TO
MEET
YOUR GOD

"Christ in you, the hope of glory."
Col 1:27

Glenn A. Pearson

PREPARE TO MEET YOUR GOD

Scriptural Meditations for the Terminally Ill and Their Caregivers

Glenn A. Pearson

Genesis Press
Lincoln, Nebraska USA

Prepare To Meet Your God
Scriptural Meditations For The Terminally Ill And Their Caregivers
By: Glenn A. Pearson

Permission for wider usage of this material can be obtained through: **www.preparetomeetyourGod.com**

Library of Congress Control Number: 2006938229

Publisher's Cataloging-in-Publication
(Provided by Quality Books, Inc.)

Pearson, Glenn A.
    Prepare to meet your God : scriptural meditations for
the terminally ill and their caregivers / by Glenn A.
Pearson.
        p. cm.
    Includes bibliographical references.
    ISBN 978-0-9765222-1-8
    Original ISBN 0-9765222-1-7
    ISBN 978-0-9765222-2-5 (audiobook)

    1. Terminally ill--Religious life. 2. Terminal care
--Religious aspects--Christianity--Meditations.
    3. Death--Religious aspects--Christianity--Meditations.
    I. Title.

BV4910.P43 2007   248.8'6175
                                    QBI06-200093

Printed in the United States of America

Cover Design by: **Nate Perry**

Ekklesia Press (and its imprint Genesis Press) are ministries to help authors get published and to publish works that are not deemed "profitable" by the mainstream publishing industry. Our goal is to put works into print that will impact and motivate followers of Christ to fulfill the Great Commission in an ever increasing way. Secondly, we want to minister to people, both Christian and non-Christian, in the way of helping them get published.

Ekklesia Press (and its imprint Genesis Press) are extensions of www.kingdomcitizenship.org

Genesis Press
Lincoln, Nebraska USA

Table of Contents

Introduction
1. Confronting Our Mortality   16
2. Prepare To Meet Your God   22
3. The Message Of The Bells   26
4. God Numbered Your Days   32
5. Life's Journey Ends With A Divine Appointment   38
6. Paradise Lost – Paradise Regained   44
7. Earthly Life Ebbing Away   52
8. The Way Of Salvation – Part I   58
9. The Way Of Salvation – Part II   64
10. The Way Of Salvation – Part III   72
11. A Time To Be Born And A Time To Die   82
12. God's Perspective On The End Of Your Life   88
13. Grace Sufficient   94
14. Character Formation Through Suffering   100
15. Simeon's Secret Can Be Yours As Well   110
16. Hand In Hand With Jesus   118
17. Pass Away – Fly Away – Departure   124
18. Setting Your House In Order   132
19. Angelic Escort On Your Trip To Heaven   140
20. Seeing The Invisible   148
21. Having The Right Kind Of Anxiety   156
22. Achieving An Attitude Of Relinquishment   164
23. What God Is Preparing For You – Part I   172
24. What God Is Preparing For You – Part II   178
25. How To Say Final Good-Byes And More   184
26. Releasing Your Loved One   190
27. Church Bells May Be Tolling   196

Appendix A   204
Appendix B   208
About the Author   212

Dedication

This book is dedicated to the glory of God, believing by faith that its contents will be a manifestation and fulfilling of 2 Corinthians 4:16, which reads; "So we do not lose heart. Though our outer nature is wasting away, our inner nature is being renewed every day." To that end, this volume is also dedicated primarily to those for whom death draws near, with the prayer that they would not breathe their last unless and until they are fully *Prepared to Meet Their God* by calling upon Jesus for the gift of salvation and eternal life. This book is also dedicated to all family members and professional caregivers as a resource for their ministry of bringing comfort and a sure hope to the dying.

Expressions of Gratitude

I will always be grateful for my wife, Esther Ruth for her indispensable gifts of encouragement, editing, and proof-reading of the manuscript again and again. My thanks are also due to Pastor Rodney Lensch who has offered wise counsel along with many prayers for the writing, publishing, distribution, and spiritual nurture for all who read its contents. My gratitude is also expressed to Kelly Haack who has edited much of this work. I am appreciative to Genesis Press and their group, who introduced me to "Print on Demand."

Foreword

As a longtime friend and colleague of Glenn Pearson, I strongly encouraged him to write this book because of his unique pastoral gifting and his rich experience in ministering to the sick and dying with divine wisdom and compassion. His credentials are impeccable.

As you will see, this book is a veritable seminar on how to face death in the faith and victory of Jesus Christ. Using Holy Scripture as his sure guide, Glenn deals with every conceivable challenge and aspect of walking through the valley of the shadow of death without fear.

At first glance, the title of this book could be misleading as if intended only for those on the threshold of death due to a terminal illness. However, its appeal is to a far larger audience for Scripture says, "Death is the destiny of every man; the living should take this to heart," Ecclesiastes 7:2 NIV. Young and old, sick and well, believer and unbeliever can all benefit from reading this much-needed volume. Since none of us knows when our date with death will occur, it behooves us all to be ready at any time. Besides, we really aren't ready to live until we are ready to die. Having dealt with the death issue, we can fully and freely get on with life.

Pastors would be wise to consider giving this book to parishioners who are senior citizens. Sometimes it is assumed that longtime church members are ready to die, when in fact they are not. When asked if they are prepared to die, they may say, "I hope so", rather than "I know so". This book will gently but firmly expose a false or weak faith and help establish a true saving faith.

My prayer is that all who read this book will be arrested by the Holy Spirit and come away with the confidence Paul displayed when he wrote: "I know whom I have believed and am convinced that He is able to guard what I have entrusted to him for that day" (2 Timothy 1:12 NASB).

Rodney G. Lensch,
Rod and Staff Ministries, Inc.
Omaha, Nebraska U.S.A.

Introduction

There is a sense in which all people of all ages are terminal regardless of whether they are vibrantly healthy, seriously ill or sick unto death. God's Word declares this sobering fact with these words: "Therefore we do not lose heart. Even though our outward man is perishing, yet the inward man is being renewed day by day" (2 Corinthians 4:16). In these modern days, many people tend to consciously or unconsciously deny this truth with an ever-increasing zeal for good nutrition, a drive for physical fitness, a quest for state-of-the-art medical care, and a variety of radical "remedies" such as cosmetic surgeries, hair replacement and the like. Nevertheless, each of us is subject to diseases, deterioration of advanced age, accidents, acts of terrorism, natural disasters, and criminals striking deadly blows. Mortality creeps up on us, or suddenly and quite unexpectedly attacks us. What then are we to do? We need to carefully focus on the positive side of 2 Corinthians 4:16 which continues to say, "Yet, our inner nature is being renewed every day." The answer to our mortality is to believe God's good news that we are more than a physical body which is destined to return to dust. We are also endowed by our Creator with both a spirit and a soul, which He promises to renew every day right up to our last day!

The primary goal of *Prepare to Meet Your God* is a daily spiritual renewal for those who are facing imminent death. An Indiana cemetery has a tombstone, more than one hundred years old, with the following epitaph:

Pause, stranger, when you pass me by:
As you are now, so once was I.
As I am now, so you will be.
So prepare for death and follow me.

An unknown passerby scratched these additional words on the tombstone:

To follow you I'm not content,
Until I know which way you went.[1]

The two-line postscript added to this epitaph makes a very wise statement. The not-so-subtle assumption is that there are only two ways we can go when we die—to Heaven or to Hell. This book will enable the dying to know with complete assurance that they can be destined for Heaven, and that the journey will commence immediately following their last breath. No one is fully prepared to die unless and until they become fully prepared to meet God before they die.

Using the Holy Bible as the primary authority for knowledge of the truth, the reader will then be led into personal experiences based on this knowledge. The end result will be an adventuresome journey with Jesus Christ through the valleys of suffering, sorrow, and death, then finally into the House of the Lord, face to face with the Living God!

Here is an important word for those of you who have acquired this book and are not totally convinced that your illness is terminal. I am fully aware that some Christians have a strong faith that their God is a God of miracles, and that sometimes these are performed for those who are at the "eleventh hour" of their life. I fully agree that God is both able and sometimes willing to demonstrate His power and love in this manner. I also believe that if Jesus would say to you, "Rise, take up your bed and go home", after having read this book you will be prepared to "Meet Your God" whenever you reach the "finish line" of this earthly life.

The back cover of a book on the subject of life-threatening disease has a caption which reads, "What to Read While Seated in Eternity's Waiting Room."[2] Being confronted with terminal illness *does* place one in eternity's waiting room! While in this "room," the Bible and the book you are holding will inspire you to hear the voice of Jesus. He will speak to you about His everlasting love, forgiveness, hope, and the gift of eternal life. By reading the Scripture passages preceding each meditation, believing the truth they express, and praying the concluding prayers, Jesus will be preparing you to die peacefully and confidently. Deep in your heart you will experience the full assurance of being prepared to meet your God.

The writings of this book are called meditations. To derive the most benefit from each message, it will be necessary to understand and practice the spiritual exercise of meditation as God ordained and set forth in the Scriptures. The content of all truly Christian meditation is the Word of God. Therefore, each meditation contained in this book is thoroughly grounded in the Holy Scriptures. The focus is always on the person of God the Father, His only Son Jesus Christ, and the Holy Spirit. Each meditation is designed to inspire the reader to be engaged by the Holy Spirit in a progressive moving from mental understanding to a dynamic experiencing of the reality of divine truth in the depths of the human heart.

Quite possibly, some persons reading this material will have varying degrees of limitation on their mental processes due to illness or advanced age. Such human frailties impose no limitations upon the Holy Spirit, who uses the Word of God to penetrate and generate within the depths of the soul a sweet mystical communion with our heavenly Father and Jesus our beautiful Savior. Godly meditation for this purpose is both God's *gift* and His *doing.* Trust Him. He will do it because His greatest desire is to experience the deepening intimacy of your love for Him as well as for you to experience the depth and transforming power of His love for you!

Some patients might possibly be too weak or lack adequate coherence to read this book and profitably concentrate on its messages. In such cases, I ask that a spouse, a family member or professional caregiver such as a pastor, chaplain, attending nurse or hospice personnel read the meditations at a pace which their patient's condition allows him/her to beneficially receive.

The meditation topics in this book are in a sequential order. Therefore, it is *not* recommended that the reader scan the various titles listed in the table of contents and make preferential choices as to which topics sound most interesting or applicable. This could result in skipping over other vitally integral meditations, all of which are important to the overall impact intended.

Words For Family Members And Caregivers

It is not uncommon for those who are entering life's final days to lapse into a partial or fully comatose state. Should this condition occur, it is helpful to know that a person in a coma is still capable of hearing sounds and comprehending conversations held in his or her immediate surroundings. This is a medical fact proven in part by studies of non-terminally ill patients who, upon recovering from their comatose state, testified that they heard and understood much of what was spoken in their presence!

Therefore, it is advised that one or more members of the care-giving team read aloud from this book to those who are in a coma. Performing this service will be exercising faith and trusting in God to richly provide spiritual edification and comfort for the dying person. Our God is mighty and will perform all that His Word declares, including daily spiritual renewal up to and especially the final day!

It is also recommended that the patient listen to audio recordings of traditional Christian hymns or contemporary praise and worship songs as another source of spiritual inspiration and strength.

[1] Ron Rhodes, *The Undiscovered Country: Exploring the Wonder of Heaven and Afterlife*, (Eugene, Ore: Harvest House, 1960).
[2] Brunvoll and Seiler, *Life on Hold, (Sisters, Ore: Multnomah Publishers, Inc., 2001).*

1

CONFRONTING OUR MORTALITY

— A REALITY CHECK —

Scripture:

Lord, make me to know my end, and what is the measure of my days, that I may know how frail I am. Indeed, You have made my days as handbreadths, and my age is as nothing before You; certainly every man at his best state is but vapor. Surely every man walks about like a shadow.

Psalm 39:4-6a

Meditation:

Unfortunately, many people the world over remain willfully ignorant, if not oblivious to portions of scripture such as the one quoted above. This is especially true during the youthful, healthful and successful seasons of life. Even during times of adversity and deteriorating health, it is highly uncommon for many individuals to contemplate or meditate on the status of their human *mortality*.

Suddenly, the *alarm* goes off. A wake-up call sounds loud and clear. But this *clock* is not equipped with a snooze button and its *shut-off switch* remains elusive. If it were a community tornado siren assaulting the ears with its wailing sounds, we would know exactly what to do: grab a flashlight, the battery powered radio and dash for the basement. However, the varied and repetitious alarms signaling our *mortality* are different! Your head physician has had the courage and professional expertise to give you the very news you may have been fearing. Using words similar to these, your doctor may have said: "Only the symptoms of your sickness are treatable; there is no known cure;" or "Your body has suffered irreparable damage from your injuries. Unfortunately, you most likely will not recover."

During the ensuing hours and days, the shock, the disbelief, and the anger, combined with a heaviness of mind and heart, will by God's grace comprise a *reality check*. This will be followed by the Lord's mercy, which will gently lead you to "teachable moments" to learn *His* Word, *His* perspective, *His* purposes, *His* plan. As you read on, the Holy Spirit will instruct you in God's truth, enabling you to accept your mortality and to be prepared to receive His *gift* of *immortality*!

Now comes the moment of truth. God is speaking to *you*! "Lord, make me to know my end and what is the measure of my days." To be strongly, yet lovingly confronted with the *brevity* of life is not bad, morbid or harsh. Why? Because God is re-focusing your life. He is about to give you a new perspective, a living hope. Listen carefully. God has more to say about human mortality. Please don't "turn Him off" because His truth is too hard to hear. The hard truth, the hurting truth in this situation is really the *healing truth*! So let it all penetrate your mind and sink deep into your soul.

His Word continues, "That I may know how frail I am." Surely the afflictions you are now bearing in your body dramatize this truth. "You have made my days as handbreadths." This bold "read out" of God's measuring rod of your longevity can be summed up in a single word: brief! "My age is nothing to You." Here's the message. The Lord has a way of swallowing up and dismissing all our temporal, chronological reckoning standards. He views all of life from His perspective of eternity. "Every man at his best state is but vapor." We need to agree! Our temporary life in this earthly body is as vulnerable as "vapor," which all too quickly *evaporates* with the heat of aging, failing health or the destructive wounds of accidental or criminal injuries. "Surely every man walks about like a shadow." At sunset shadows disappear; so it is, at the sunset of this life. It is good, in God's eyes, for us to cease being shadows and be escorted by Him into the "Light of Life". That Life is eternal life purchased for all who believe in the saving power of Christ's death on the cross. By God's grace, this book will prepare you to eventually walk into the shadow-less light of the Father of Lights (James 1:17). Begin now to lift up your eyes "unto the hills from whence

> **Man at his best state is but a vapor...which all too quickly evaporates.**

your help comes" (Psalm 121:1 **KJV**).

To know in the depths of your spirit and soul the brevity, the transience, the frailty, and the vulnerability of this life is to experience God's goodness and mercy. If you receive it as such, you will be given a new measure of *dependency* upon His grace. Now is the time to release a *heart-cry* for His mercy. With humility, plead for the Holy Spirit to focus your eyes on Jesus who is ready to give you new hope and to usher you into the glorious future He has prepared for you. Yes, in one sense your earthly life is almost over. But in a much greater sense, it is just about to begin!

Prayer:

Oh Lord, my eternal God, Thank You for Your painful, yet gracious summons to face my mortality. Please help me to come face to face with You through Your Word and Your Holy Spirit. Fix my gaze upon Jesus and strengthen my hope, faith and love for You. In His Name. Amen.

I HAVE FOUND THAT
ENDURING PAIN,
WHETHER PHYSICAL,
EMOTIONAL OR SPIRITUAL,
MUST OFTEN BE
DONE IN SILENCE.
IT IS A LONELY VIGIL, BUT
ONE THAT THE SAVIOR
UNDERSTANDS AND
SHARES WITH YOU.

— Judson Cornwall —

From: *Dying With Grace*, pg. 65-66

PREPARE TO MEET YOUR GOD

Scripture:

Therefore thus will I do to you, O Israel; because I will do this to you, prepare to meet your God, O Israel.

Amos 4:12

Meditation:

"Prepare to meet your God," that is what this book is all about. Though we are created in the image of God, possessing spirit and soul as well as a mortal body, death inevitably will come. When death does come or when Christ returns to earth, the first thing that will happen is that we will meet God face to face, one on one. What an ominous encounter that will be! What a dreadful experience awaits all who die unprepared to meet their God! What an *awesome* experience awaits those who are truly *prepared* to meet their God!

"I have faced terminal illness... this is a special time to confront my fears..."

Judson Cornwall, a mighty man of God, who, having served Him for 70 years as a preacher, teacher, counselor, and prolific author, was diagnosed with prostate cancer and given only three months to live. However, he lived with this death-sentence prognosis not just for three months, but for three years! He gave the following testimony: "I have faced terminal illness every day. Yet I've learned that this is a special time to confront my fears, challenge my doubts and trust my heavenly Father."[1] This book, by God's grace, and by the power of His Word and Holy Spirit, will help you do the same, regardless of the number of days, weeks or months remaining in your life.

When I was a lad growing up in rural Wisconsin,

there was a county road with a particular type of road sign that, over the years, never faded, rusted, or tilted. Rather, it stood tall with its singular, direct, and powerful message, "Prepare to Meet Your God." Usually, I rode in the back seat of our family auto and liked to watch for this sign. As always, it would loom up and grab my attention. Without questioning the truth of it—after all, it was taken from the Bible—I did wonder what it meant to "meet" God and what one should do to be prepared for such a meeting. The sign always left me puzzled because I knew so little about "meeting" God and even less as to when, where, and why it might happen to me.

The book you are reading is intentionally designed to hold before you several times and in a variety of ways the same message: "Prepare to Meet Your God." You will be instructed in practical and specific ways how to be prepared. Most of the following meditations will focus your attention on certain scriptures, which deal directly with both the meaning of and the tasks necessary for an encounter with your loving Creator.

After your death, there will be no time or opportunity to make preparations. Now is the time to seek the Lord and learn from His Word about the care and counsel of your Good Shepherd, Jesus Christ.

Be assured that Jesus will manifest His presence to you during the pain and afflictions of your circumstances and your physical condition. Through the grief and sorrow of bidding farewell to your family and other loved ones, God Himself will enable you to experience His supportive love. This love will be poured into your heart by the Holy Spirit in answer to your prayers and those of your loved ones. Also included in this care will be the team of medical professionals ministering to your medical needs. Dear friend, God is preparing to meet you right where you are and just as you are!

Prayer:

Father in Heaven, I thank and praise You for Your unconditional and unfailing love for me. Thank You for the knowledge that You desire to meet with me these days before I die. Help me, I pray, to humbly submit to making all the necessary preparations in my heart and soul to meet You face to face. Please remove all my fears, and kindly assist me to fully cooperate, and to make the most of Your divine encounters with me. In Jesus' Name. Amen.

THE MESSAGE OF THE BELLS

Scripture:

And upon its hem you shall make pomegranates of blue, purple, and scarlet, all around its hem, and bells of gold between them all around. And it shall be upon Aaron when he ministers, and its sound will be heard when he goes into the holy place before the Lord and when he comes out, that he may not die.

Exodus 28:33, 36

Meditation:

In the course of a life, different bells with many different messages register in our ears, our heart, our mind, and our memory. There are school bells, dinner bells, ship's bells, shore bells, cow bells, boxing bells, fire bells, storm bells, clock bells, and, of course, church bells. Each bell has its own message.

Before there were church bells, there were tabernacle and temple bells. These bells, as described in the scripture quoted above, were initially part of the Levitical priestly garments. The message of these vestment bells was twofold. First, the bells were intended to be a continual reminder to the priest who wore the holy garments that wherever he went he was in the Holy Presence of the Lord. Second, these bells gave a message to the worshiping community that the priest had entered into the holy place to make atonement for his sin and for their sin. Moreover, the bells assured the worshipers that the high priest had made it out safely, thus signifying that the sacrifice he offered was pleasing and acceptable to God.

Centuries later, church bells were elevated from priestly garments to high steeples and/or carillon towers. The purpose was to allow the bells to signal the faithful to assemble in the sanctuary, much like the school bells ring out the message that recess is over and classes are about to resume. Church bells were also sounded in the hope that the clarion tones reverberating in a several-mile radius would summon folks with no church affiliation to be a part of the *community gathered for worship.*

Historically, cathedral and church bells were and still are sounded in different ways on different occasions. Church bells are rung resoundingly on the Lord's Day and other days announcing times of worship. Church bells are rung joyfully on wedding days or at other times calling for celebration such as the victorious end to a war.

In the church of my childhood in rural Wisconsin, the huge and high steeple bell could be heard for miles. It was always joyfully rung at the climax of a New Year's Eve service of fellowship and worship. Several minutes before midnight, the old year was "rung out." At the precise twelve o'clock hour the New Year was "rung in."

Many church bells, and other large bells, are also equipped with a side-mounted lever-action clapper designed to generate a quite different sound known as the toll. The tolling of the church bell produces a somber, rather mournful sound. In this manner, it is used at the conclusion of a funeral or memorial service. The message of the church bell when tolled has a very clear impact. Death is saddening, sorrowful, resolute, and final. Tolling church bells stir the emotions and command respect for the life and service of the deceased. I liken it to the impact and purpose of "taps" or a rifle salute at a military funeral.

This brings me to share a story from the life of the English poet and preacher John Donne (1572-1631). He tells of the time of his illness, which led to his death. Donne's home was in close proximity to a large cathedral with a high steeple equipped with a loud bell. He relates how again and again that cathedral bell tolled death after death. Though he had a deep respect for this traditional practice, the repetitious tolling eventually became an irritant to his soul. It was not so much the dissonance of the toll sound as the message it kept "pounding" home. Stated in his own words, "Now, this bell tolling softly for another, says to me, 'Thou must die.'"

John Donne went on to tell about the common community response whenever cathedral or church bells were tolling: "I wonder for whom the bell is tolling now?" This inquiry prompted the poet's very profound and oft-quoted response: *"Therefore, never send to know for whom the bell tolls; it tolls for thee."* [1]

I have chosen to call all who read the meditations of this book "my friends." So, my friend, are you receiving the message of the tolling bell? Will you allow your imagination and your memory to reverberate afresh until it really grips your soul? If so, let it do so while its message penetrates as deeply as necessary to quicken your mind and heart to hear with all sincerity God's vital Word to make "all things well with your soul." God is seeking to capture your respectful attention, like blasting cannons honoring the dead who heroically served their country in the armed forces.

> Church bells stir the emotions and command respect for the life.

Your funeral or memorial service may or may not be held at a church with a steeple bell. In any case, tolling bells or none; know that your passing will sound a "bell-being-tolled message" to many. Your family, relatives, friends and persons of the community in which you lived need the same sort of dramatic reminder of their own mortality that God has granted you.

Prayer:

Lord God of Heaven and earth, I need to know that You are the God of the living and the dead. I celebrate with thanksgiving all the *ringing* bells, which I have heard throughout my life. Help me now to hear and accept the real and symbolic *tolling* of the church bell, as closure to my life approaches. I have heard from your Word that there is going to be a wonderful wedding in Heaven between You Jesus, my Bridegroom, and me as a cherished member of Your corporate Bride. Inspire me to anticipate hearing the joyful *ringing* of those wedding bells. Help me during the remaining days of my life to be fully prepared to be wedded to You forever! In Your Holy Name, Jesus, I pray. Amen.

[1] John Donne, "Meditation XVII," *Devotions Upon Emergent Occasions* (New York: Random House, Inc, 1952), used by permission.

GOD NUMBERED YOUR DAYS

Scripture:

Your eyes saw my substance, being yet unformed. And in Your book they all were written, the days fashioned for me, when as yet there were none of them.

Psalm 139:16

Since his days are determined, the number of his months is with You; You have appointed his limits, so that he cannot pass.

Job 14:5

Meditation:

No doubt you have heard the fairly common saying referring to the time of a person's death, "When your time is up, it's up." But do you know that this saying is taken from the Bible and represents a paraphrase of Psalm 139:16 quoted above? God *does* determine the life span of every individual while still developing in the womb. All persons created by God have been given a free will. This, in part, is what it means to be made in "the image of God." Unfortunately, many unwise free-will choices expressed repeatedly in destructive life-style patterns significantly abbreviate a divinely appointed life span. Some examples would be the use of tobacco, abuse of drugs including alcohol, and compulsive over-eating. Likewise, the failures and sins of other individuals, as well as corporate segments of society, rob many persons of the length of days God intended for them to enjoy.

Be that as it may, God is never "behind" when it comes to all the necessary revisions He must make regarding His chronological bookkeeping of our days and years. God is totally omniscient—knowing all things—so He is never "surprised" by having to make changes from His *projected* longevity to your *actual* longevity, which He fully knows you will experience. This is true because the Bible declares our God to be "The Alpha and the Omega, knowing the end from beginning" (Revelation 1:8).

The God who numbered your days while you were yet in the womb, is the same God who has also been numbering the very hairs of your head throughout your lifetime (Matthew 10:30). Jesus declared this as a reality! In this instance, He was *not* speaking figuratively. He also said, "Not one sparrow falls to the ground apart from your Father's will." Amazing! If God both *knows* and *wills* the death of a single sparrow, most assuredly He knows the day and the hour of your death (Matthew 10:29). If God so cares for each sparrow, how much more will He continue to infinitely care for you during these difficult days of facing death? This providential care will be expressed by purposefully and completely preparing you to meet Him on that very day!

God earnestly desires to "Teach us to number our days, that we may gain a heart of wisdom" (Psalm 90:12). The deeper meaning of this passage is not merely to keep a chronological record of our age. We don't need to be taught how to do that! Jesus has a greater concern, which is to teach us that He measures our life span in days, not years. Truly, this is another summons to be lovingly confronted with the reality of our own impending last days well in advance of *the* last day!

How good and gracious of God to promise that He will teach us to "gain a heart of wisdom." You might very well be asking, "What is the purpose of seeking to gain wisdom now after my life is almost over?" It really takes much wisdom from above to live a God-pleasing life. Even more so, it takes much wisdom, which only Jesus can give, to be prepared to pass *through* death and stand in the presence of a Holy God. The remaining meditations in this book are designed to teach you Biblically based wisdom about dying and thus prepare you to meet your God. More importantly, you will be guided into an *experiential application* of this wisdom of the heart, which is totally relational. This means that the purposes of the Lord for your remaining time on earth are to have you be exclusively devoted to a deeper and more intimate relationship with Him. His desire is

> God earnestly desires to teach us to number our days.

for you to be fully assured that He is so willing, so able, so eager and so ready to clasp your hand and "lead you through the valley of the shadow of death and into the house of the Lord to dwell in His presence forever" (Psalm 23). Are you ready to trust Him totally for a fearless and awesome adventure far beyond anything this earthly life has offered you?

Prayer:

Thank You, my Father, for creating me with a destiny and purpose, which has only begun during my earthly life. Jesus, I humbly ask You to teach me the wisdom only You can give, to prepare me for eternity with You. Please remove my fears and doubts, which rob me of faith. Help me trust that You have grasped me with Your right hand and will escort me into the heavenly home You have prepared for me. Thank You, Holy God, for Your goodness and mercy, which have been following me all the days of my life. In Jesus' Name I pray. Amen.

SO TEACH US
TO NUMBER OUR DAYS,
THAT WE MAY
PRESENT TO THEE
A HEART OF WISDOM.

Psalms 90:12
NASB

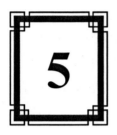

5

LIFE ENDS WITH A DIVINE APPOINTMENT

Scripture:

And as it is appointed for men to die once, but after this the judgment.

Hebrews 9:27

Meditation:

Life lived in these modern times tends to be an uninterrupted series of appointments. Many of them are of our own choosing; some are not. The feverish pitch and pace of contemporary life demands fancy daily planner books. Some very busy people utilize high-tech mini computers called Palm Pilots or Blackberries. Even cell phones and laptop computers now come equipped with daily planning options and are being used by business persons, professionals, and even common folk, all of whom are busily on the run, needing to keep track of daily appointments and their "to-do" list.

As Christians, we need to be reminded that God has both the desire and the right to call us for personal appointments to meet with Him. These meetings are called *divine appointments,* and rightly so. "You shall remember the Sabbath Day to keep it holy." That was, and still is, a divine summons to meet our Creator and Redeemer for worship *at least* once a week. Our God desires us to keep regular appointments with Him for prayer, reading His Word, and as guests at His table to commune with Jesus by partaking of His Holy Supper. Even in your weakening condition, it is not too late to make a wholehearted effort to keep some of these divine appointments. For His sake and your own sake, give it your very best!

These are just a few of the times and circumstances that the Lord has planned for regular appointments with Him. To be sure, God is busier than any of us mortals, running the universe and caring for every creature in Heaven and on earth. Yet He is never too busy to keep His appointments with each one of us and to graciously respond to all our needs.

However, such is not always our response pattern. Regarding the activities and meetings logged in our daily planners, we find it necessary at times to reschedule our appointments. At other times, calls are made to cancel the appointment, along with excuses for doing so. Occasionally, no communication is offered and the appointment is broken by just not bothering to "show".

> God has the desire to call us for appointments.

Periodically, this same pattern "spills over" into keeping our divine appointments as mentioned above. We all must be reminded that there is one major exception. Hear it again from God's Word: "It is *appointed* for mankind once to die, but after this the judgment" (Hebrews 9:27). [Emphasis added] Be very certain and fully persuaded that this is one divine appointment which is inevitable, inescapable and unbreakable! Considering your medical diagnosis, you already know that your closing days are approaching. Being reminded of this may seem to be somewhat heartless or even cruel, until you begin to meditate on the truth that your own dying process and death itself is an appointment with God! Possibly, this appointment may sound to you like a threat, some sort of a "trip to the wood shed" for stern dealings with God. Continue reading and learn that the exact opposite is true.

Dear reader, whoever you are, whatever your background and your beliefs, know that your appointment with the Lord has already begun. Be prepared for an awesome experience. More than that, it is also God's gracious intent to make it an altogether beautiful experience. As you give Him your undivided attention, He invites you to fully give Him your mind, your heart, your emotions, [including anger if it is present], your doubts, and your fears. He is your Father! He has no desire to threaten, intimidate or corner you. He does not, and will not, withhold His mercy, His forgiving love, and His all-sufficient grace. In such a loving encounter, do not hold back anything from Him! Pour out your heart to Him. Confess any secret sins and seek earnestly to come to a full acceptance, a complete surrender, and a sweet resignation of your whole being to Him. He deserves nothing less! Jesus is present to comfort and help you. He desires that you embrace your closing days as a sacred time, a godly closure of your earthly life!

Prayer:

Dear God, my Father: I acknowledge that I have been stirred and challenged by Your word to me in this meditation. I admit that I am not fully comfortable with this divine appointment experience. But I want to embrace in my heart all You have to say and to do all You require of me. I ask for Your help. Thank You for not leaving me now when I need you the most! In Your mercy, hear my prayer offered in Jesus' Name. Amen.

WHEN I DISCOVER
THE LORD ON HIS TERMS,
I WILL BE ABLE TO LET GO
OF MY OWN WORRIES
AND CONCERNS
AND SURRENDER TO
HIM WITHOUT ANY
FEAR OF PAINS AND
SUFFERINGS...

— Henri Nouwen —
From: *The Genesee Diary*, pg. 159

6

PARADISE LOST

PARADISE REGAINED

Scripture:

And they heard the sound of the Lord God walking in the garden in the cool of the day, and Adam and his wife hid themselves from the presence of the Lord among the trees of the garden. Then the Lord God called to Adam and said to him, "Where are you?"

Genesis 3:8-9

Meditation:

Walking is perhaps the simplest form of exercise and yet the most beneficial. Walking *with* God is the best of all therapies for the body, soul, and spirit. It was God's idea to have routine strolls with Adam and Eve during the cool of the evening in the beautiful Garden of Eden. It was literally a perfect paradise. All the species of trees, shrubs and flowers were created and planted by God Himself! Adam and Eve were totally sinless and knew how to enjoy God's holy presence without fear. Having not yet fallen from their perfect state of innocence, their marriage undoubtedly was filled with the same blissful splendor of an evening stroll in "the park" with their Creator God who was revealing Himself as their intimate *friend*!

Suddenly, on one fateful day during one fateful hour, their free choice to remain perfectly content and fulfilled without the "knowledge of good and evil" was tested. The devil, in the form of a serpent, slithered into the garden, having chosen to seduce Eve. As the "father of all lies," his strategy was to introduce Eve and Adam—in that order— to the greatest lie that would ever be told to the human race! Essentially, Satan's deception went like this— "You will never be happy or truly fulfilled until you eat from the forbidden tree and become *like God,* possessing all knowledge of good and evil."

The renowned Christian author, John Milton (1608-74), in his epic poem *Paradise Lost,* told "Of man's First disobedience and the Fruit Of that Forbidden tree whose mortal taste Brought death into the world, and all our woe, With Loss of Eden" (Book I - 1-4). All that happened in the moment Adam and Eve believed the lie and disobeyed God's commandment and committed the sin of death. Milton composed a sequel to this book and entitled it *Paradise Regained that told of Christ's coming.* Yes, Adam's and Eve's sin did result in the loss of their innocence, causing them to immediately experience shame and guilt. Not only did *they* fall into sin; their deliberate act of disobedience plunged the whole human race into the horrible legacy of being born with a sinful nature. King David, upon committing back-to-back sins of adultery and murder, in the time of his shame and guilt confessed: "Behold, I was brought forth in iniquity, and in sin my mother conceived me" (Psalm 51:5).

> Walking with God is the best of all therapies for the body, soul and spirit.

We need to listen carefully to what God spoke to

Adam and Eve when He confronted them with their blatant act of disobedience. While He did pronounce a curse upon both the *devil* and the *ground*, He did *not* curse Adam and Eve. Yes, God did declare that they would suffer serious consequences of their sin, but He did not curse them!

Many who learn that their sickness *is* going to lead to death find this thought crossing their minds—is my death a curse from God? For some this thought does not merely *cross* their minds, it continues to *plague* their minds! Do not let the devil lie to you as he did to Adam and Eve! Rather, welcome the Lord as He ministers grace to you as He did for Adam and Eve. Grace extends the peace and comfort of knowing that although sin against God does break beautiful *fellowship* with Him, but His *relationship* with those who are guilty is not *severed*!

The unfolding story in Genesis dramatically demonstrates God's mercy and grace. After Adam and Eve's Fall, the Lord came seeking the ashamed and guilty couple. His ultimate goal was to restore the rich fellowship of the garden rendezvous. "Adam, where are you?" Of course God knew where they were! No one can ever hide from God. Once you grasp the abundance of His grace, you will *never* again try to hide from Him! God knew exactly behind which trees Adam and Eve were cowering in shame. He called out to let them know He was actually *seeking* to restore their broken fellowship; He was not angrily rejecting them because of their disobedience. Do you get the picture? It is God, prompted by unconditional love, who takes the *initiative* to restore through forgiveness and recon-ciliation our broken fellowship with Him. Thus begins the Gospel story of redemption for you and me who, no less than Adam and Eve, begin to *regain the paradise* of the new Heaven and the new earth symbolized by the Garden of Eden.

A second major adventure beautifully illustrating God's plan for paradise regained follows. Adam and Eve tried to cover up the shame of their nakedness by making garments from fig leaves. What a feeble attempt at a covering! How long would it take for plucked fig leaves to wither and crumble in a hot tropical climate? "The soul that sins shall die" (Ezekiel 18:4). Here is the lesson: all attempts to become self-righteous by seeking to compen-sate for sinful disobedience through good deeds (including religious good deeds), will surely crumble in the "hot climate" of God's judgment.

This beautiful Gospel account recorded in Genesis proceeds to declare *God's way* of covering Adam's and Eve's guilt and shame. How about leather garments hand-tailored by God Himself? Quite a contrast from shriveling, crumbling fig leaves! "And the Lord God made for Adam and his wife garments of skins, and clothed them" (Genesis 3:21). From this account we learn that the blood and sacrificial death of these animals represent a foreshadowing of the shed blood and death of Christ on His cross. No other religion in the whole world is able to offer *this only acceptable sacrifice* ordained by our Holy God granting forgiveness, removing shame, guilt, and condemnation. "For He made Him who knew no sin to be sin for us, that we might become the righteousness of God in Him" (2 Corinthians 5:21).

What an awesome expression of the Gospel according to Jesus! Right now He is offering you faith to *believe* and receive His very own righteousness as a garment to wrap around your soul. If you humbly say, "Yes Jesus, I desperately need Your perfect righteousness," you will receive that righteousness and thus be prepared to stand in His presence unashamed and guilt free, ready to step into the eternal paradise created for you!

It is true! Paradise is indeed regained by the gift of God's only begotten Son. Jesus Christ freely paid the penalty of our sin by His sacrificial death for you, for your loved ones, and for all who will completely trust in Him alone for their eternal salvation. No sins of thoughts, words or deeds (past, present or future), which are confessed to Jesus, will keep anyone out of God's paradise in Heaven. This paradise far surpasses the beauty and grandeur of the Garden of Eden, which was but a picture of the one to come!

Remember what Jesus spoke to the thief who also was being crucified. Near the hour of his death he earnestly pleaded, "Jesus, remember me when You come into Your Kingdom." To this humble and simple request, Jesus quickly replied, "Assuredly, I say to you, *today* you will be with Me in Paradise" (Luke 23:43). [Emphasis added]

Prayer:

Thank You, God, for walking with me in the many beautiful garden-like experiences of my life. I acknowledge that You have also been calling out to me in those times of my stumbling, and my falling short of Your glory because of my sin. Now I sincerely believe that all the while You have been seeking to find me and to draw me to Yourself. Forgive me, Oh Lord, for all the times I have rebelled and chosen to walk alone among the thorns and thistle patches of this earthly life. Jesus, I praise You for thinking of me and remembering me as You took my place on the cruel cross. Please, be very close to me on the day of my death. In Your mercy, escort me all the way into Your paradise prepared for me. In Your Holy Name I pray. Amen.

7

EARTHLY LIFE
EBBING AWAY

Scripture:

And God has reserved for His children the priceless gift of eternal life; it is kept in Heaven for you, pure and undefiled, beyond the reach of change and decay. And God in His mighty power, will make sure that you get there safely to receive it, because you are trusting Him. It will be yours in that coming Last Day for all to see. So be truly glad! There is wonderful joy ahead, even though the going is rough for a while down here. These trials are only to test your faith, to see whether or not it is strong and pure. It is being tested as fire tests gold and purifies it—and your faith is far more precious to God than mere gold; so if your faith remains strong after being tried in the test tube of fiery trials, it will bring you much praise and glory and honor on the Day of His return. You love Him even though you have never seen Him; though not seeing Him, you trust Him; and even now you are happy with the inexpressible joy that comes from Heaven itself. And your further reward for trusting Him will be the salvation of your souls.

I Peter 1:4-9[1]

Meditation:

Through 38 years of serving the Lord as a pastor, I have frequently used this scripture to bring comfort, courage and hope to those whose time of departure to go home to be with the Lord drew near. As you meditate and reflect upon these divine words from God Himself directly given to you, I am sure your faith will be strengthened. Jesus is the giver and sustainer of all having true faith in Him. Through this time of testing, His purpose is only to increase your faith, which will enable you to endure the pain and the many discomforts you are experiencing these days. During this time of great need, the Lord will empower you to grow in your ability to become increasingly dependent upon Him. He is your only source of strength as your own ability to cope is rapidly depleting.

The Bible tells us in many places that God our Father is our stronghold. This truth refers not so much to our strong hold on Him, as to His strong hold on us! His powerful hand has had a grip on you all your life. Surely, He will not let you slip out of His hands nor out of His everlasting arms in this your time of great need! Here is another wonderful promise from His Word, which will counsel and comfort you: "You will keep him in perfect peace, whose mind is stayed on You, because he trusts in You" (Isaiah 26:3).

His strong desire is for you to experience a full measure of His love.

The many and unique hardships you are daily and hourly facing, are the ultimate test of your faith. One more promise from your heavenly Father: "No temptation has overtaken you except such as is common to man; but God is faithful, who will not allow you to be tempted beyond what your are able, but with the temptation will also make the way of escape, that you may be able to bear it" (1 Corinthians 10:13). The Greek word translated "tempted" in this passage can also be interpreted accurately to mean "tested". Jesus is the way of escape referred to. Stay focused on Him by drawing upon His strength and He will *build* your faith. Rest assured, He will not allow your faith to be stretched to a breaking point. Instead, His strong desire is for you to experience a full measure of His love, which "bears all things, believes all things, hopes all things, endures all things" (1 Corinthians 13:7).

Prayer:

My God, my Father: In the strong Name of Jesus, I call upon You, to offer my praise and thanksgiving for Your Fatherly care which supplies all of my needs for all my remaining days. Thank You for not allowing me to be tested beyond my strength. And I thank You that with the tests You will provide the way of escape that I may be able to remain faithful until the end. Thank You for always hearing my prayers as well as those of my family and friends. Please bless all my doctors, nurses, and caregivers. Give them Your wisdom to be expressions of Your unfailing love to me and to one another. Thank You, Jesus, for being my good and faithful Shepherd, leading me to Your "green pastures" and "still waters" even in this time of great suffering. I ask these things in Your Holy Name. Amen.

[1] Holy Bible, *New Life Living Translation,* (Wheaton, IL: Tyndale House Publishers, Inc., 1976).

SWIFT TO ITS CLOSE
EBBS OUT
LIFE'S LITTLE DAY;
EARTH'S JOYS GROW DIM,
ITS GLORIES PASS AWAY;
CHANGE AND DECAY
IN ALL AROUND I SEE;
O THOU WHO
CHANGES NOT
ABIDE WITH ME!

— **William H. Monk** —
From: *Abide With Me*
Stanza 2, Public Domain

8

THE WAY OF SALVATION PART I

Scripture:

And where I go you know, and the way you know. Thomas said to Him, "Lord, we do not know where You are going, and how can we know the way?" Jesus said to him, "I am the way, the truth, and the life. No one comes to the Father except through Me."

John 14:4-6

Meditation:

This meditation and the two

following are the most *crucial* of all the meditations in this book. If you are already a Christian, having experienced a spiritual rebirth, these three meditations will serve to *reaffirm* your faith based on a complete trust in Jesus as your personal Savior and Lord. If you are not certain about your spiritual readiness to be received by God and welcomed into His Heaven when you die, these meditations will clarify for you what it means to *receive* Jesus, *believe* in Jesus, and to be *born again* into His Kingdom.

> Jesus alone *personifies* and *embodies* the way, the truth, and the life.

Thomas was an amazing guy! He was one of the twelve apostles chosen by Jesus. For three years, he had been taught by Jesus, the master of all teachers. Yet, when Jesus announced the approaching time of His Ascension back to His Father in Heaven, Thomas was confused, puzzled, and full of questions. He asked: "Jesus, where are you going? What is the way?" Speaking on behalf of the other eleven apostles, he said, "We don't know the way. How can we know the way?"

We shouldn't be too quick to criticize or judge this man. Many individuals of our time have been raised in Christian homes by godly parents, taken to Sunday school and church services. As adults they have attended church for years. And yet, they are much like Thomas, not really knowing with full *assurance* what it means to follow Jesus and to have a personal relationship with Him based on trusting faith alone.

It has been said, "If you want the right answers, you have to ask the right questions." We have to give Thomas credit for being on the "right track" with his honest questions! True to His manner of teaching, Jesus replies with the *right* answer, speaking directly and simply. "I am the way, the truth and the life. No one comes to the Father except through Me."

With the direct statement, "No one comes to the Father except through Me," Jesus, for all time, swept away all falsehood, misunderstanding, and confusion regarding the way of salvation. Contrary to mountains of doctrinal error and many popular opinions, together with the insatiable drive for religious inclusiveness in our modern society, Jesus boldly declared, and continues to declare that there are not many roads, acceptable religions, systems of philosophy or self-righteous good works leading to reconciliation with the heavenly Father. There is only *one* way, and Jesus Christ alone is that way! There are *no* exceptions, *no* alternatives, *no* other gods, and *no* other saviors!

With one fell swoop Jesus denounces and dismisses all religious inclusiveness and calls for a new mindset of exclusiveness for all would-be believers desiring to follow Him *alone.* There are but two responses one can make to this bold declaration of a *single* way to the Father. You can take offense and stumble over Jesus' exclusive declaration and dismiss it as narrow mindedness and judgmental religious bigotry. Or you can be very grateful to Jesus for His profound *simplification* of the way of salvation. God grant you the faith and courage to take the holy highway and follow the one way of Jesus that leads to eternal life!

Allow me to add one more clarification of Jesus' assertion "I am the way, the truth and the life." When Jesus prefaced His statement with the words "I am", He proclaimed that He alone *personifies* and *embodies* the way, the truth, and the life. It is a common practice of many to reduce the Christian faith to abstractions of theology, dogmas, doctrines, creeds, and rituals. These each have their place in teaching and propagating divine truths *about* Jesus. But they must never become a substitute for a personal, deep, and intimate relationship *with* Jesus who is the risen Lord, and who is alive forever more. The essence of such a relationship is trust expressed in open and honest interpersonal communication with your only Savior. He is your best friend. He already knows you, and your deepest needs and desires. As you completely trust in Jesus, the Holy Spirit will draw you into a joyful fellowship with Him. You will experience the inner witness of the Spirit who grants you full assurance that you possess God's *gift* of eternal life! "The Spirit Himself bears witness with our spirit that we are children of God" (Romans 8:16).

Prayer:

Lord Jesus Christ: I want to praise and thank You for coming to me in my hour of desperate need. I humbly ask You to draw me to Yourself. In Your mercy, deliver me from pain, doubts, confusion, and fear. Please lead me to Your Father and my Father. Help me, I pray, to truly embrace You as my way, my truth, and my life. Truly, I long to rest secure in

Your loving arms. In Your blessed Name, dear Jesus,
I pray. Amen.

9

THE WAY OF SALVATION PART II

Scripture:

He was in the world, and the world was made through Him, and the world did not know Him. He came to His own, and His own did not receive Him. But as many as received Him, to them He gave the right to become the children of God, to those who believed in His name: who were born, not of blood, nor of the will of the flesh, nor of the will of man, but of God.

John 1:10-13

Meditation:

Get ready to thank and praise Jesus for teaching the way of salvation so clearly! At the outset, He was clear about there being only one-way leading to the Father. With that sharp focus on Jesus as our premise, I will now present more clear teaching about specific steps to becoming born again. Entering into God's plan of salvation is really quite simple. Essentially, He is saying, "If you will take two *simple* steps toward Me, I will take one *major* step toward you, and your eternal salvation will be accomplished!"

Your first step is to *receive* Jesus. Your second step is to *believe* in Jesus. According to the teaching of John in the text quoted above, *both* receiving Jesus and believing in His Name are essential to becoming a "child of God" and being "born again into His Kingdom". These two key words—receiving and believing are deeply inter-related, but they are not synonymous! Receiving Jesus is essentially a decision to become *relationally* involved with Him by asking Him to come into your *heart*. Believing in Jesus is essentially a decision to continuously yield your *mind* to becoming a disciple who obediently follows His will and His ways. Our God whole-heartedly responds to these decisions with His giant step of accomplishing in you a spiritual rebirth into His Kingdom. Please read carefully and ponder deeply as this two-step entry into a saving relationship with Jesus is further explained.

Chapter one of John's gospel records two kinds of public responses to Jesus' beginning ministry. "He came to His own [His own people—the Jews] and His own did not receive Him" (John 1:11). Note that their negative response was their refusal to receive Him. By rejecting Jesus as their Messiah, they rejected His truth and in the process rejected the salvation He came to bring them! The second response John describes was a positive one. The positive response focuses on a remnant that did receive and believe in Jesus.

> Your first step is to *receive* Jesus. Your second step is to *believe* in Jesus.

"Receiving Jesus," means to accept the person of Jesus as your very own personal Savior. You do this by faith, making a humble decision to invite Him to come into your heart and to take up permanent residence there. One of Jesus' other names is

Immanuel, which means "God with us" (Matthew 1:23). Jesus is truly God. He is also truly man, having taken upon Himself our human form. The good news is that the burning desire of Jesus' heart is to be so much *with us* that He earnestly seeks to dwell *in us.* Right now is the time for you to take this first step.

A most blessed experience immediately follows a decision to receive Christ into your heart; it is the God-given capacity to *believe* on His Name. This is the second step God asks you to take. The word "believe" as used in the Bible has an important double meaning. First, it is a positive *mental* response, which fully agrees with the truth Jesus teaches and embodies. Second, this kind of believing is demonstrated by a sincere willingness to follow Jesus in *active obedience* to His Lordship in the values and the priorities of daily life as set forth in the Bible. This is what the scriptures refer to as believing with the heart. "If you confess with your mouth the Lord Jesus and *believe in your heart* that God has raised Him from the dead, you will be saved. For *with the heart one believes* unto righteousness, and with the mouth confession is made unto salvation" (Romans 10:9-10). [Emphasis added]

If by simple child-like faith, you take these two steps of receiving Jesus personally into your heart and making a commitment to believe in His name, you are thereby prepared to experience the greatest of all God's miracles, which is being born again by the power of the Holy Spirit. Listen to how the Bible speaks of this spiritual rebirth: "But as many as received Him, to them He gave the right to become children of God, to those who believe in His name: who were born, not of blood, nor of the will of the flesh, nor of the will of man, but of God" (John 1:12-13).

Nicodemus, a Pharisee, a teacher and a "ruler of the Jews", came secretly during the night to have a private interview with Jesus. He initiated the conversation by commending Jesus on His ministry of miraculous signs and wonders. Jesus' immediate response was to steer Nicodemus away from miracles performed in public to the personal miracle of miracles; namely, being born again spiritually. Jesus said to him (and says to all of us), "Most assuredly, I say to you, unless one is born of water and the Spirit, he cannot enter the Kingdom of God" (John 3:5).

Permit me to paraphrase and amplify what Jesus

teaches about being born again. "Make no mistake about it, Nicodemus, I'm telling you the absolute truth. You, and no one else in the whole world, including all generations, will ever get into Heaven without being born again. Your parents only gave you a physical birth. The second birth, which you must experience, is spiritual. It is exclusively the work of the Holy Spirit giving new birth to your spirit, which is dead as a result of your sins and transgressions. Nicodemus, I know you are not able to receive this teaching because of many unanswered intellectual questions of your natural mind. Know this for sure: spiritual rebirth is a mystery that goes far beyond the ability of your finite mind to comprehend."

Here is an illustration. There are many mysteries occurring in the natural world, like the wind. Tell me, do you know where it comes from or where it goes? No, you don't! In the same way, there are many mysteries in the spiritual world of God's Kingdom. Your inability to understand them doesn't make them any less real. If you agree to allow God's Spirit to give you a spiritual rebirth, you will have a new mode of knowing spiritual truth, and will begin to experience dramatic changes in your life. Yes, Nicodemus, being born again in your spirit by the power of the Holy Spirit is very real!"

I hope my paraphrase was helpful. Nicodemus walked away from this private session with Jesus having failed to meet His challenge to become born again into the Kingdom of God. His stumbling block was his spiritual pride based on high learning about all the religious traditions of Judaism. *However,* we do know according to John's testimony (John 19:39), that at some point in the course of Jesus' three-year public ministry, Nicodemus did become a true believer and follower of Jesus.

What about you, dear friend? If you have never personally received Jesus into your heart, *now* is the time. You probably don't have much remaining time to humbly yield your total being to Him. He is your God, having created you. He is your Lord and deserves your trust and service for all eternity to come. As your Savior, Jesus laid down His life for you on the cross. His blood, shed for you and all sinners, is the *only way* to receive forgiveness of all your sins, past, present, and future. Only Jesus can cleanse you and clothe you with His perfect righteousness. Without the justification that results from being made righteous, no one is acceptable to our Holy God.

In conclusion, permit me to ask you a very important question. Is not your Father God who created you, and His only Son, Jesus, who sacrificed Himself for you, and the Holy Spirit who offers to give you a spiritual rebirth, worthy of a positive response by humbly receiving the free gift of eternal life? You may give God your positive answer by sincerely praying the prayer, which follows.

Prayer:

Dear Lord Jesus: I come to You confessing that I am by nature sinful and unclean; and that I have sinned against You by thought, word, and deed. I need to be saved. I desire to be born again. Jesus, I receive You by faith. Please come into my heart to forgive and to cleanse me from all sin and unrighteousness. I yield my spirit, my soul, and my body to You. Lord Jesus, with all my heart and mind, I truly want to believe in You and be Your loving friend and Your faithful servant. Thank You so very much for loving me, and freely giving me Your gift of salvation and eternal life. In Your mercy, hear my prayer, which I offer in Your most Holy Name. Amen.

10

THE WAY OF SALVATION PART III

Scripture:

For by grace you have been saved through faith, and that not of yourselves; it is the gift of God, not of works, lest anyone should boast. For we are His workmanship, created in Christ Jesus for good works, which God prepared beforehand that we should walk in them.

Ephesians 2:8-10

Meditation:

Part one of this three-part series of meditations on the way of salvation placed a sharp focus on Jesus as the *only* Savior. The salvation He brings is everlasting peace with God and full assurance of citizenship in His eternal Kingdom of Heaven. Part two made clear the proper *response* to His offer of a free gift of eternal life, which is to personally *receive* Jesus and trustingly *believe* in Him with both heart and mind. This basic commitment leads directly to the spiritual experience Jesus called being *born again* into the Kingdom of God. This third meditation develops some of the initial Kingdom of God dynamics characteristic of the Christian life.

It is so refreshing to know that eternal life is a *quality* of life that unfolds as a beautiful flower here and now. All sense of guilt and shame are gone, replaced by the peace and joy of knowing with complete assurance that your destiny with Christ and the glorious company of saints and angels is *settled* and *sealed* by His precious blood. On this point, God's Word unequivocally declares this truth: "These things I have written to you who believe in the name of the Son of God, that you may *know* that you have eternal life" (1 John 5:13). [Emphasis added] The meaning of the word "know" in this passage is to know by virtue of an intimate relationship with Christ. Many sincere persons striving to live the Christian life to the best of their ability, when asked if they know for sure that they will go to Heaven when they die, reply by saying, "It is impossible to know that for sure in this life. You will just have to wait and see what happens on judgment day." How terribly sad! Hopefully, this is not your testimony. Should you not be fully confident of being Heaven-bound upon your death, more faith-building, Scriptural teaching follows.

> Have I done enough good works to offset my sinful deeds and tip the scale in my favor?

The Apostle Paul was quite genuinely concerned that the Christians in the city of Ephesus clearly understood the foundational truths of life with Christ. "For by grace you *have been saved…*" (Ephesians 2:8). [Emphasis added] Note carefully that salvation is an accomplished fact for these believers, and it is God's own doing which is by grace alone. The term "grace" as used in the Bible means, essentially, undeserved mercy. The best example of salvation by grace alone is the thief on the cross next to Jesus. He came to a truly repentant attitude realizing that Jesus was his only hope to escape a deserved   destiny of Hell. He said, "Jesus, remember me when you come into your kingdom." Jesus' reply was: "Assuredly, I say to you, today you will be with Me in Paradise (Luke 23:43). This amazing response must have astounded him! In addition to receiving full assurance of his salvation, Jesus promised him a place with Him in Paradise. Perhaps the majority of persons reading this book have only one thing in common with this criminal—the reality of death drawing close. Yet, many others, and perhaps you are one of them, are in desperate need of an "eleventh-hour" crying out to Jesus for His forgiveness of your sins leading to the same gift of salvation by *grace alone*.

More reassuring good news comes later in this same passage of Ephesians. Salvation is "not of works, lest anyone should boast (Ephesians 2:9). The world is filled with religions. All of them, with the single exception of true Christianity, teach that mankind is capable of performing a multitude of "good works" which merit salvation. The primary motivation for doing these religious good works is to demonstrate self-righteousness, moral acceptability and personal character worthy and deserving of admission to God's Heaven. Such teaching is completely false and generates a false sense of security for salvation. A performance-based hope for salvation results in a lifetime of nagging uncertainty. "Have I done enough good works to offset my sinful deeds and tip the scale in my favor of being judged worthy of Heaven and not deserving of Hell?" Hear me! Reject the lie. Believe only what God says. The only good work that will admit you or anyone else into Heaven is the work of Jesus' sacrificial death on His cross coupled with His mighty Resurrection on the third day! Salvation is not for sale. It cannot be earned or deserved. Why? Because it is a free gift of God's mercy and grace through Christ. Jesus said, "You shall know the truth, and the truth shall make you free" (John 8:32). So let God's truth set you free from trusting in any form of good works you have done, leading instead to complete faith in Christ's good work for *you* on His cross.

There is yet another exciting principle of life in the Kingdom of God. Interesting enough, it has to do with the good works God has prepared for you as His loving servant. What a holy honor God bestows upon all His children, born again and fully alive in His Spirit! He calls us "His *workmanship* who have been created in Christ Jesus for good works which God prepared beforehand that we should walk in them" (Ephesians 2:10).

As you know, this world is filled with gifted and talented artisans. Some are highly skilled, some semi-skilled, but all possessing a measure of skill adequately equipping them to do the specific good works He has assigned for them to do. Most artists, technicians and workers of many trades, take pride in their respective workmanship, and rightly so. Think how much more pride our heavenly Father takes in us who are His workmanship! In this manner, He confers dignity, meaning, and fulfillment upon all, who in any capacity, serve Him.

Possibly you are wondering why I'm discussing good works, which God has prepared beforehand for us to do. I have two reasons. The first is to affirm you in the Name of the Lord for the good works you have done throughout your lifetime serving Him and others. Listen as He speaks to you: "For God is not unjust to forget your work and labor of love which you have shown toward His name, in that you have ministered to the saints, and do minister" (Hebrews 6:10).

My second reason is to speak of God's good work prepared for you in the hereafter. Now is the time to gain eternity's perspective on your divine destiny in the new Heaven and the new earth that God is going to create. As God's special workmanship, it is not too soon to joyfully anticipate what you are about to experience when you "report for duty" on your new "heavenly good works" assignment! Maybe you have some regrets for not being more zealous and enthusiastic about rendering good works for the Lord and others during your life. Perhaps, on the other hand, your employment circumstances may have caused you to live with frustration because of lack of more meaning, fulfillment, joyous reward or financial gain. Possibly you kept going from job to job searching for your niche in life, but somehow it always eluded you. In modern society there are many disgruntled workers who, if they don't speak it loud, keep nurturing the attitude expressed by the words, "Oh hell, it's Monday" and "Thank God it's Friday"!

Dear friend, if in any measure this mindset describes you and your past circumstances, I say, "God's peace be unto you!" Dismiss the regrets. Let the negative emotions discharge. Allow frustration to drain away. Cast off the heavy weights of purposelessness and disappointment. Take heart—Jesus' heart. These days are now all but over. Your Lord God is about to purge you, as may be necessary, of this "gunk". Your new eternal good works assignment fully prepared by God awaits you. This job is full time. The pay will be far greater than you can spend. No computer spreadsheet can display all the benefits. No need to wonder about a promotion. You will be at the "top" from the very beginning. You will be more than pleased with your "Employer". His pleasure with you will be unending.

Are you receiving this message? Believe it! It is not merely fanciful, wishful or wistful. Quite the contrary, these truths are reality talk based on biblical revelation. Here is just one example: "These are the ones who come out of the great tribulation, and washed their robes and made them white in the blood of the Lamb. Therefore they are before the throne of God, and *serve Him day and night* in His temple. And He who sits on the throne will dwell among them" (Revelation 7:14-15). [Emphasis added]

A concluding postscript: since, as stated above, doing good works can never earn or repay God for His gift of eternal life, what should be our proper motive for being eager to joyfully do the good works God assigns to followers of Jesus both here on earth and in the age to come? The answer in a single word is *gratitude*! Our hearts cannot but overflow with gratefulness for all the grace and mercy poured upon us in the Beloved Redeemer—Jesus Christ! This never-ceasing heartfelt attitude of thanksgiving to the Triune God is delightfully rendered by us through worship and work (which, for the Christian, are synonymous and equally sacred) both here and in the hereafter.

Prayer:

Dear heavenly Father: my heart is stirred and my mind is being renewed by all the inspirational truth of Your holy Word. Humbly, I ask You to quicken all this revelation concerning the way of salvation to become living and active in my daily life. I love You for loving me even while I was a sinner. My desire is to be eternally grateful for Your forgiveness of all my sins, and for Your gift of my salvation. Words cannot express the love and joy I have in You. So I thank and praise You for making me Your divine workmanship, and preparing good works suitable for me to perform. From the depths of my heart, I long to see You face to face, and to feel Your strong embrace. With gladness and joy, I look forward to worshiping You and serving You with the clean hands and the pure heart You have given me. Holy Father, I pray in the mighty Name of Your Beloved Son, Jesus. Amen.

11

A TIME TO BE BORN AND A TIME TO DIE

Scripture:

To everything there is a season, a time for every purpose under Heaven: a time to be born and a time to die... He has made everything beautiful in its time.

Ecclesiastes 3:1, 2, 11

Meditation:

When you were born, it occurred in God's time. He chose your parents; He chose your generation, and your time in history. You were God's perfect gift to your parents, your grandparents, and to any brothers and sisters you may have had at that time. You were created with talents, gifts, abilities, purpose, and destiny. Your God made you and the "time and season" of your birth to be beautiful! Your creation and birth were His doing. It gave Him pleasure. In Genesis 1:31 it is written: "Then God saw everything that He had made, and indeed it was very good." Accordingly, on the day you were born, God looked at the person He had made and said it again: "This is very good."

Be assured that these same truths regarding the *time* of your birth all equally apply to the *time* of your death! As your health gradually gives way to illness, you are doubtless receiving much medical care, many visits, greeting cards, phone calls, and prayers offered to God Almighty on your behalf. As you continue to experience all this loving support, be assured that your Lord is making all things to work together for your good as promised in His Word (Romans 8:28).

Obviously, there are many seemingly insurmountable hardships attending these closing months, weeks, and days of your life. Yes, you are very likely experiencing pain that is pushing past your medication as your body wastes away. And yes, there is the emotional pain associated with preparing for the severance of life-long relationships with those whom you dearly love, and who dearly love you. There is also the mental pain attending all those unanswerable questions. Why me? Why now? Why so soon? I'm not that old yet! Or, Why all these prolonged days, weeks, months, or maybe even years of suffering? Finally, there is also the spiritual pain expressed in questions like these: Why, God? Why are you cutting me off?

During these times of severe afflictions, prayerfully ask the Holy Spirit to comfort you with the knowledge that Jesus is fully empathizing with you. On this point, God's Word assures you: "For we do not have an high priest which cannot be *touched with the feeling of our infirmities*; but was in all points tempted like as we are, yet without sin" (Hebrews 4:15 **KJV**). [Emphasis added] Jesus is that High Priest; and He has experienced, to the greatest possible degree, the very same forms of physical, mental, and spiritual anguish on His cross. From there He cried out, "My God, My God, why

> Now is the time to cling to your loving Heavenly Father with complete trust .

have You forsaken me" (Matthew 27:46). Just one or more of these types of pain would seemingly be enough to contradict and refute all the above declarations of "God making death beautiful."

However, now is the time to cling to your loving heavenly Father with complete trust and dependence. Doing so will enable you to rest in the promises of His Word. The result will be His perfect peace gradually washing away negative feelings, unanswerable questions, and doubts. Here is one example of the powerful promises God has declared for this time of preparing to meet Him face to face as death draws near. "Who shall separate us from the love of Christ? Shall tribulation, or distress, or persecution, or famine, or nakedness, or peril, or sword? For I am persuaded that neither death nor life, nor angels nor principalities nor powers, nor things present nor things to come, nor height nor depth, nor any other created thing, shall be able to separate us from the love of God which is in Christ Jesus our Lord" (Romans 8:35; 38-39).

When you were born, it was traumatic for you, and painful for your mother. During your infancy and toddler years there were pains and stressful difficulties. Yet God made these moments beautiful in His time. Surely He will faithfully fulfill all the promises His word declares. As you reflect upon your life, do you not see in retrospect God's goodness and mercy attending you through all the seasons of life? Has He once failed you in the midst of pain, adversities, uncertainties and questionings?

Now is the time to trust God more deeply and completely than ever before. Even the *capacity* to trust Him more implicitly is itself His gift to you. Trust and faith are His "tools" to fashion your death to be beautiful in His eyes. While I was serving as senior pastor to a congregation in Woburn, Massachusetts, the choir director from time to time would select a particular anthem to be sung at funeral services. The anthem contained the following profound lyric: "Thou, Oh Lord hast made death beautiful and triumphant for through its portals we enter into the presence of the Living God!"[1] What a beautiful expression of the truth of His Word: "You have made everything beautiful in its time" (Ecclesiastes 3:11). The all-inclusive *everything* in this passage includes the dying experience.

So, my friend, here is my pastoral counsel to you. By God's grace, completely yield to Jesus your family and all your loved ones, your pain, your sorrow, your heartache, your questions, your fears, and all doubts. He will take all these hurts and anxieties and make them beautifully redemptive!

Keep your expectation alive. There are yet more "gems" and much fine "gold" that He has prepared to unearth for you in the meditations to follow. Please keep reading, keep meditating, and keep praying. Your heavenly Father will do everything else to make the closing time of your life beautiful. He is faithful. He will do it!

Prayer:

Mighty God, Everlasting Father: Thank You for stretching my faith and increasing my trust in Your love and power. Please make the time of my death beautiful just as You have promised. As I have been seeking to live for Your glory, help me also to die for Your glory. Perform a miracle! Make my remaining days and my hour of death a testimony of Your saving grace that will inspire and bless all my loved ones and friends. In Jesus' Name, I ask these things. Amen.

[1] Will C. Macfarlan, "Open Our Eyes" (New York, NY – G. Schimer, Inc., 1928).

12

GOD'S PERSPECTIVE ON THE END OF YOUR EARTHLY LIFE

Scripture:

Precious in the eyes of the Lord is the death of His saints.

Psalm 116:15

For My thoughts are not your thoughts, nor are your ways My ways, says the Lord. For as the Heavens are higher than the earth, so are My ways higher than your ways, and My thoughts than your thoughts.

Isaiah 55:8-9

Meditation:

It will be easier to draw upon the comfort of God's grace and mercy if you allow Him to show you His perspective on the death of His saints. To do so enables you to think His higher thoughts and to follow His higher ways, leading directly into His Kingdom of everlasting life. The tender mercies of God will allow you to shift from *your* temporal worldview to *His* eternal worldview. Be confident! Your Lord is able to open your spiritual eyes and enlighten your finite mind to actually see what He sees and think what He thinks. As this happens, your impending death will begin to become as precious to you as it is to Him!

> Earthly struggles and sickness will have given way to heavenly rest and peace.

Here is how God's higher worldview applies to Christians who are in the process of this great transition. Preparing to say goodbye to loved ones for the last time, as difficult as it is, becomes somewhat easier as you begin to anticipate saying hello to Jesus face to face for the very first time. Note that Psalm 116:15 is addressed exclusively to "His saints". The Biblical use of the term "saints" is defined as persons whose sins are forgiven because they truly believe in Jesus as their Savior. Death is precious in God's eyes because it is the "threshold" which must be crossed to be initiated into this most glorious transition.

I shall try to speak about this transition experience in simple and yet profound terms. It is to go from bodily death to a full experience of divine life. It is to leave the earth having been set free from a diseased, pain-racked body. It is to be ushered into the presence of Jesus. It is to bid farewell to your loved ones remaining on earth and to be welcomed "home" by your fellow saints and the angels. It is to experience a thrilling family reunion with believing loved ones who preceded you on this heavenly journey. It is to make the profound spiritual shift from *trusting faith* in God and Jesus to the *magnificent sight* of the realms of glory. Earthly struggles and strife, sorrows and sickness will have given way to heavenly rest and peace. Dear friend, these are just a few reasons why "Precious in the eyes of the Lord is the death of His saints!"

Back to earth—right now, your death in your own eyes without this heavenly vision and hope would be quite the opposite of precious. It is almost always painful in virtually every way pain can be experienced. It is often fearful. You may be feeling lost and lonely, shrouded in the fog of mystery, uncertainty, doubts and insecurity. Perhaps you are somewhat bereft of spiritual reality in general, and of the belief in life after death in particular. If this describes your present frame of mind in any way, I trust God's Word, which is like a fire, will burn away this fog and clear the way for you to receive God's higher thoughts and higher ways about your imminent future with Him!

You are precious to the Father and to Jesus His Son. That's why your coming to faith and trust in Him and eventually going to Him on the day of your death is so precious in His eyes! Even now, He is drawing you nearer to Him relationally. This reality brings Him much joy. He waits longingly to draw you all the way to Himself and to His Son Jesus and the heavenly abode, which He has prepared for you. Your sovereign God is in control. His great desire is for you to humbly yield to Him so that He can make your death precious in *your* own eyes just as it is already precious in His eyes!

Prayer:

My Lord and my God, I believe. Help me to escape all my unbelief. Keep inspiring me to think Your higher thoughts and walk Your higher ways so clearly revealed in your Word. In Your loving kindness, gently wean me from earth and prepare me for Heaven. Allow me to feel Your precious touch in all my many hurts. I need You. I desire You. Please increase my faith to humbly come to You as a child. I pray in Jesus' Name. Amen.

WHERE DEATH IS AFFIRMED, HOPE FINDS ITS ROOTS.

— Henri Nouwen —

From: *The Genesee Diary*, pg. 78

13

GOD'S GRACE SUFFICIENT

Scripture:

And lest I should be exalted above measure by the abundance of revelations, a thorn in the flesh was given to me, a messenger of Satan to buffet me, lest I be exalted above measure. Concerning this thing I pleaded with the Lord three times that it might depart from me. And He said to me, "My grace is sufficient for you, for My strength is made perfect in weakness."

2 Corinthians 12:7-9

Meditation:

It is most unlikely that there is much similarity between the Apostle Paul's experience of heavenly revelations and our more limited grasp of divine truth. To keep Paul from spiritual pride, God allowed Satan to afflict him with an unspecified infirmity. In the course of time, Paul sensed this physical malady to be a definite handicap to the success of his missionary calling. He pleaded with the Lord three times to be delivered from this demonic intrusion into his life and ministry. God had a surprisingly different answer to his prayer. Instead of the thorn being removed, Paul was promised that God's all-sufficient grace would compensate him far and above his perceived inability to fulfill his apostolic mission in life. He was told by the Lord that His powerful grace would be made perfect in his weakness.

> I believe the Lord's message to you is... My grace is entirely sufficient for you!

The word of the Lord may have been something like this: *Paul, I know how to handle whatever the devil and the human condition can throw at you and make it work powerfully for My purpose for your life.*

My grace will cause you to become increasingly dependent upon Me and thus My work through you will be perfected. My grace will enable you to endure the hardship of your malady and effectively accomplish your ministry at the same time. Trust Me, my son, your labors for Me will not be haphazard, but will have the mark of excellence and complete accomplishment.

Dear friend, your serious illness may be the result of not one, but several "thorns" in your flesh. After much prayer and the best treatment modern medical technology has to offer, the thorns may remain and maybe they are beginning to fester. Perhaps they are becoming toxic not to only your body, but your mind and your spirit as well. What to do now?

Personally, I believe the Lord's message to you is similar to what He spoke to Paul. I believe He would call you by name and say, "My grace is entirely sufficient for you! I am preparing you to be ready to meet Me face to face. My grace for you is the complete assurance and the peace of knowing that I have clothed you with the robe of My righteousness. Even as your physical body is gradually wasting away, I will cause you to rest in the knowledge that you are Mine, now and for eternity to come. During the time remaining for you on earth, My grace will make you strong even in the midst of pain and sorrowful heartache. Continue to trust Me, and I will give you strength to endure and even cause you to be a witness of my perfect love to those around you."

Now would be a good time for you to meditate upon the thorns in the flesh, which Jesus endured as part of His suffering passion to save you. It was not just two or three thorns, but a full circle of braided thorns forming a mocking crown. The crown was not gently placed on His head, but crushed down upon it like an ill-fitting cap.

Doubtless, a stream of blood flowed down His sacred head from each piercing thorn. With both hands nailed to the cross, it was not possible for Him to thrust off this instrument of torturous pain. With complete dependence upon His Father's grace, Jesus endured the excruciating pain, and especially the horrific agony of being forsaken by His Father God. Please know with certainty that Jesus is fully acquainted with the pain of the thorns in your flesh and the anguish of your soul. Your knowing that Jesus completely identifies with your suffering will strengthen you to face your pain, anguish, and sorrow with the same sustaining grace that enabled Him to face His death. Undoubtedly, your weakness is increasing. Nevertheless, His grace flowing upon you is fully sufficient. Be confident that it will increase day by day according to your need. God's Word promises, "As your days, so shall your strength be" (Deuteronomy 33:25). Cast all your cares upon Jesus, knowing that His loving care for you will never end.

Prayer:

Lord Jesus, I confess that I truly need every measure of sustaining grace You have to offer. I thank You for giving me the strength to endure the pain of the "thorns" in my body. Though they are not removed, I am grateful to You for removing the "thorns" of shame, guilt, fear, and even anger toward You in my spirit and soul.

Thank You for replacing the weakness caused by these thorns with the strong graces of Your love, forgiveness, hope, and peace. Dear Lord, I thank You for Your loving compassion, which fully identifies with my sorrow and pain. You wore and bore the crown of thorns in order that I might wear Your crown of righteousness. For these, and all Your mercies and grace, I will remain eternally grateful. In Your Holy Name I pray. Amen.

14

CHARACTER FORMATION THROUGH SUFFERING

Scripture:

Therefore, having been justified by faith, we have peace with God through our Lord Jesus Christ, through whom also we have access by faith into this grace in which we stand, and rejoice in the hope of the glory of God. And not only that, but we also glory in tribulations, knowing that tribulation produces perseverance; and perseverance, character; and character, hope. Now hope does not disappoint, because the love of God has been poured out in our hearts by the Holy Spirit who was given to us.

Romans 5:1-5

Meditation:

Please allow me to ask you a personal question regarding your spiritual life: do you have any hope? Have you any hope for today, for tomorrow, for the future, which will transcend your death? We who teach God's Word sometimes speak too abstractly about spiritual life. The goal of this meditation is to address the basics of Christian faith as they deal with the practical issues of daily life. What characteristics does God look for in the person seeking spiritual maturity? The answer is found in 1 Corinthians 13:13: "And now abide faith, hope, love, these three; but the greatest of these is love."

What a simple and yet profound statement! Who but God speaks like that? Note carefully, God measures spirituality primarily in terms of character virtues. Some Christians tend to emphasize two different standards of measuring spirituality. One is good Biblical knowledge *about* God coupled with experiential knowledge stemming from a personal relationship *with* God. The other is performance of good deeds. Jesus' teaching clarifies how *both* sound doctrine and performance of good works, which God has prepared for each individual believer, are complementary and necessary in the development of Christian maturity and virtuous living.

Listen carefully to this sobering teaching by Jesus: "Not everyone who says to Me, 'Lord, Lord,' shall enter the Kingdom of Heaven, but he who does the will of My Father in Heaven. Many will say to Me in that day, 'Lord, Lord, have we not prophesied in Your name, cast out demons in Your Name, and done many wonders in Your Name'? And then I will declare to them, 'I never knew you; depart from Me, you who practice lawlessness' " (Matthew 7:21-23).

For what reason will these many well-informed and power-driven "followers" of Jesus be judged unfit for the Kingdom of God? What standard of judgment will Jesus use? The answer is found in His phrase, "I never knew you." Here is the truth we *must* grasp. Character virtues cannot be effectively imparted without a deep interpersonal relationship with Jesus!

This truth applies equally to other interpersonal

relationships as well; for example, the relationship of husbands and wives who are also parents. Frequently, they become too busy to spend quality time getting to know their children. In some cases, parents tend to be strangers to their children's unique personalities, hurts, and desires. They are, in fact, too busy to effectively impart the godly character virtues children so desperately need. Keep in mind that God our Father and Jesus our Wonderful Counselor are never too busy to spend time getting to know us! The truth is they already know us better than we know ourselves! Therefore, any failure to develop an intimate relationship with our Lord is entirely our own shortcoming. Even so, God in His merciful grace has ways of drawing us out of our lesser preoccupations and bringing us to an "on-our-knees" dependency upon Him. This completes the necessary groundwork to address the specific theme of this meditation, which is character formation through suffering.

➢ Let us turn back to my original question about your level of hope. Three primary character virtues I referred to are faith, hope, and love. Of these, hope is the central focus of this meditation. For purposes of illustration, I will use a candle as a symbol for hope. Do you have a candle of hope? Perhaps you once did, but it's been consumed by burning long days and longer nights as you've been struggling to cope with the strains and pains in your body coupled with the mental stress of unanswered questions and doubts. Your candle of hope is but a stub, too short to light one more time! Or perhaps the candle is only partially burned. It keeps getting snuffed out by a succession of increasingly serious symptoms of your illness. All these cruel realities flooding upon you may have depleted the willpower to relight your candle of hope. Perhaps you are begin-ning to realize that your candle of hope doesn't have even a flicker. It's out!

> I will use a candle as a symbol for hope. Do you have a candle of hope?

If the negative aspects of the analogy I have just described apply to you very little or not at all, praise and thank God. But if the "down side" does apply, it is time to praise and thank God in this situation as well! Returning to Romans chapter 5, Paul talks about two *types* of hope, which God supplies. They are distinct and contrasting. First is the "hope of glory" to be realized in Heaven to come. The second way God transforms our character into the image of Christ is the "glory produced by tribulations" during our earthly life. This heavenly hope of glory, which God richly supplies, burns more brightly than the sun and is cause for great rejoicing. The Bible declares God to be the *God of all hope*. This means that God is the source of all hope, which never disappoints, fades, falters, or fails. All forms of hope emanating from God are anchored in the bedrock of His Word.

This hope of His glory is twofold. First and foremost, it is the hope of being totally conformed to the *image of Christ*. Think of it! God has actually begun to infuse us with His divine sinless nature in this life. This sacred transformation is a continuing process, which will be fully and finally consummated in the life to come. Pause and think about the implications of this miraculous wonder! We will no longer have even any taint of a sinful nature. We will never sin again because every trace of our *capacity* to sin will have been totally obliterated forever! Isn't that a truly glorious hope and cause for great rejoicing? A Scriptural definition of this hope reads as follows: "And I am sure that God who began the good work within you will keep right on helping you grow in this grace until His task within you is finally finished on that day when Jesus Christ returns" (Philippians

1:6)[1]

ᵛ God has a variety of ways to transform our character to the image of Christ. We will focus on just one of His ways, one which seems strange and even contradictory to our way of thinking. Paul teaches that Christians are to *glory in tribulations.* Tribulations take many forms and assault the believer in a variety of ways. Some of them are persecutions resulting from publicly confessing our faith in Jesus as Lord. Other forms of tribulation are poverty, wars, famine, disease, and eventually death itself. Strange as it may seem to our way of thinking, God actually does *use* hardships, afflictions, and suffering to forge and impart character transformation into believers who trust Him for the gift of eternal life.

Listen again to the manner in which tribulations generate specific character virtues in Christians. Three are mentioned in this order: *perseverance, character and hope.* Note that hope itself is identified as a primary godly virtue. It is not just a futuristic expectation of receiving the other greater virtues. Hope is the backbone which upholds, strengthens and sustains the many other Christ-like traits that God develops in us. Hope is God's gift of a solid grip on life no matter what it "dishes out," including sickness unto death! God's gift of hope manifests itself as a stubborn determination to not give in, give up or be mastered by any set of circumstances. Hope from God fuels the drive to press in and press on until His promises are fulfilled and victory is thereby fully assured!

Dear friend, your loving Father God wants you to know that *all* the suffering, sorrow, and brokenness of heart you are experiencing as you endure to the end has a *redemptive purpose!* This statement is based on the Word of God recorded in Romans 8:28-29 which proclaims: "And we know that *all* things work together for good to those who love God, to those who are the called according to His purpose. For those whom He foreknew, He also predestined to be *conformed to the image of His Son,* that He might be the firstborn among many brethren". [Emphasis added] Yes! God does work character formation through suffering, and for sure this includes the suffering leading ultimately to the end of life on earth.

The second part of God's hope of glory is His desire for us to become firmly anchored in His promise of a new and glorious *body.* The Book of Revelation declares many things about Heaven, what it is like, and what those who go there will   experience. "And God will wipe away every tear from their eyes; there shall be no more death, nor sorrow, nor crying. There shall be no more pain, for the former things have passed away" (Revelation 21:4).

Since God gives the gift of everlasting life and has abolished death forever, that can only mean one thing. He shall clothe our spirit with a new body, which will remain fully alive forever! The former things regarding our temporal earthly body will have passed away. Our new and glorious body will totally transcend things like disease, sickness, infirmities, old-age deterioration and vulnerability to injuries. How shall God's Heaven-bound saints be clothed with such a body and by whom? Answer: *Jesus!* He said, "I am the Resurrection and the life. He who believes in Me, though he may die, he shall live. And whoever lives and believes in Me shall never die" (John 11:25-26). Do you believe this? If you do believe this, your candle of the hope of glory will burn brightly and not be overcome by the darkness of physical pain in your body or by emotional sorrow in your soul! Accordingly, may God grant you the desire and capacity to rejoice in the hope of the glory of God, which is Christ in you. This hope will not disappoint you "Because God's love has been poured out in our hearts by the Holy Spirit who was given to us" (Romans 5:5).

Prayer:

Dear heavenly Father: I ask You for a greater measure of trust and faith to believe and to receive all the truths of this meditation. I truly need these truths to become living and active within me. Forgive me, if I have allowed pain and suffering to produce distrust and anger. Please replace the whole range of these negative emotions with the gifts of Your character virtues. I need and desire this miraculous transformation within the depths of my soul. Thank You for Your perfect love that enables me to "bear all things, believe all things, hope all things, and endure all things" as promised in your Word. In the Name of Christ my Savior I pray. Amen.

---

[1] Holy Bible, *New Life Living Translation*, (Wheaton, IL; Tyndale House Publishers, Inc., 1976).

15

SIMEON'S SECRET CAN BE YOURS AS WELL

Scripture:

And behold, there was a man in Jerusalem whose name was Simeon, and this man was just and devout, waiting for the Consolation of Israel, and the Holy Spirit was upon him. And it had been revealed to him by the Holy Spirit that he would not see death before he had seen the Lord's Christ. So he came by the Spirit into the temple. And when the parents brought in the Child Jesus, to do for Him according to the custom of the law, he took him up in his arms and blessed God and said: "Lord, now You are letting Your servant depart in peace, according to Your word; for my eyes have seen Your salvation which You have prepared before the face of all peoples, a light to bring revelation to the Gentiles, and the glory of Your people Israel."

Luke 2:25-32

Meditation:

In this heart-warming narrative from the infancy of Jesus we see how God blesses and uses servants who are "just and devout," joyfully awaiting the coming of the Messiah in the person of Jesus. Simeon was elderly and in his latter years. What a comforting and exhilarating secret word he received from the Holy Spirit. I choose to call it a "secret" because this revelation came to no other devout Jew besides Simeon. This promissory word was: "Simeon, you are not going to see death until you have first seen the Lord's Christ." That would be none other than the child Jesus!

Dear friend, quite possibly you have been living a just and devout life, not unlike Simeon. Now that your death is imminent, the Holy Spirit desires to comfort you in the same way He comforted Simeon. Soon it will be possible for you to see Jesus—not as a baby, but as the King of kings and the Lord of lords. Jesus, your best Friend, is waiting to see you face to face!

On the other hand, perhaps you are one who has lived a good life, but have never experienced a personal relationship with Jesus. Take heart! The Holy Spirit has a personal revelation for you also. His message for you is this: before your death takes place, you too can embrace Jesus as the One who loves you with everlasting love. He gave His life on the cross for you. If you are willing, just like Simeon, you can experience a spiritual embrace with Him in your heart. Now!

Listen as Jesus declares to you that He has already accomplished the forgiveness of your sins. His desired response is to hear your humble invitation for Him to come into your heart as your very own Savior and Lord. If you will sincerely extend this invitation, God promises that the time will indeed draw near for you to embrace and be embraced by Jesus upon your arrival into the glorious heavenly kingdom He has prepared for you.

This will take place immediately following your final breath!

Certain Christian denominations observe a special liturgical order of worship whenever the service includes the celebration of Holy Communion. Upon completion of the distribution of the Lord's Supper, the entire congregation rises to sing the "*Nunc Dimittis*" which is a Latin phrase meaning "now departing". The words of this song are a direct quote from Simeon's prophecy: "Lord, now You are letting Your servant depart in peace, according to Your word; for my eyes have seen Your salvation which You have prepared for all peoples."

> Our God is the God of our dying no less than He is the God of our living.

Perhaps you are becoming a bit unsettled with my frequent use of the "D" word (death) in these meditations. I make no apologies for that because the word "death" is the most common word found in scripture with reference to both the physical and spiritual termination of life. However, the Bible does have another softer and more profound and theologically correct word for death. That word is "depart". It describes the imme-diate separation of the human spirit from the deceased body. The next meditation will develop this truth and provide practical applications. Pay close attention to the words and grammar of Simeon's declaration. He says, "Now You are letting Your servant depart in peace, according to Your word." Simeon wasn't asking God for a departure (please let me die). Rather, he was affirming that right now God was granting his desire to depart from this temporal life. Moreover, he believed that it was to be a *peaceful* departure.

Simeon's faith enabled him to confess that there would be no fear, no anxiety or haunting doubts about his preparedness to die and face the unknown "beyond the veil". Yes, Simeon's secret can and should be ours as well. Likewise, his comforting prophecy should prompt us to confess that: "Our God is the God of our *dying* no less than He is the God of our *living.*" How good and gracious He is at all times and in all circumstances, especially when we need Him the most!

A concluding word about Holy Communion. It is altogether appropriate for believers to leave the altar, and conclude the worship service singing,

"Lord, now let your servant depart in peace." In this setting, the reference is not so much to dying as it is to living a life of peace and meaningful service in the community where the Lord sends His servants as they leave the sanctuary. The same truth has a direct application to you, since you are about to leave the sanctuary of your body and be escorted to the heavenly sanctuary to join the ranks of His saints who are *serving* Him night and day.

Of course, I do not know about your personal beliefs and participation in the Holy Communion experience. But I do highly recommend that you avail yourself of the opportunity to partake. Jesus, on the eve of the Passover Feast, said to His disciples gathered in the Upper Room, "With fervent desire I have desired to eat this Passover with you before I suffer" (Luke 15:22). Surely, Jesus fervently desires to have Communion with you by offering you the Bread of His body broken, and the Cup of His blood shed. By accepting His gracious invitation to be His guest for this sacred meal, you will be sealed by the Blood of the New Covenant, which will convey to you the blessed assurance of a peaceful departure from your earthly life.

I recommend that you request to receive Holy

Communion from your pastor. If you are currently not under the care of a personal pastor, feel free to contact a hospital or nursing home chaplain and request a visit to your bedside for private Communion. I am confident that such professional caregivers would be pleased to minister pastoral care in the form of scripture reading and prayers as well as Communion. At the conclusion of this ministry you can, by faith, make the same declaration as Simeon: "Lord, now You are letting Your servant depart in peace." For in the partaking of the Body and Blood of Christ, you have indeed embraced Jesus the Messiah, whose sacred *Presence* is so beautifully manifested in the Communion He instituted.

Prayer:

Thank You, Lord, for teaching me that my death will not be the "end of me." Help me to fully trust You for a peaceful departure leading me in my spirit directly to You and the heavenly dwelling You have prepared for me.

Please grant this blessed experience to me also. I bless You for Your gift of Holy Communion. May I participate in this most sacred fellowship with You? As I suffer physical pain daily, nightly, and hourly, keep me ever mindful of how much You suffered on the cross for me and for all sinners. Thank You for Your complete forgiveness and for a peaceful departure for my heavenly home. Holy Father, please give ear and heart to my cry offered in Jesus' Name. Amen.

16

HAND IN HAND WITH JESUS THROUGH DEATH'S SHADOW

Scripture:

Yea, though I walk through the valley of the shadow of death, I will fear no evil; for You are with me; Your rod and Your staff, they comfort me.

Psalm 23:4

Inasmuch then as the children

have partaken of flesh and blood, He Himself likewise shared in the same, that through death He
might destroy him who had the power of death, that
is, the devil, and release those who through fear of
death were all their lifetime subject to bondage.

Hebrews 2:14-15

Meditation:

Very likely the strongest of negative emotions
that came rushing upon you when you learned of
your terminal condition was the fear of death. Fear
always accompanies the unknown. For this reason,
everyone fears death because it remains an unknown to all who have not experienced it. Jesus,
having experienced the most horrible form of death,
and having totally triumphed over it, is your
greatest of all needs. He has a strong desire to be
everyone's perfect pastor. He said, "I am the Good
Shepherd." The term "shepherd" in the Hebrew
language is synonymous with the more contemporary term "pastor."

Jesus is perfect in everything He has done and
continues to do. What makes Him the perfect pastor
is the fact that through His incarnation He is both
true God and true Man. He took upon Himself our

human form and faced death head on. He did more than just *endure* it. He actually *conquered* death by destroying him who has the power of death—the devil! Therefore, as the Hebrews text declares, Jesus has the power to *deliver* us from our life-long bondage to the fear of death. He doesn't just help us to cope with the fear of death; Jesus completely removes and delivers us from the fear of death. If we humbly submit to Him, He will set us free from this demonic bondage! This He does for all believers, vibrantly healthy or sick unto death.

Dear friend, if you are not completely free from the fear of your death, reach out to Jesus and by faith receive His perfect love afresh this very moment. In 1 John 4:18, God's Word declares that "perfect love casts out fear." The purest expression of this perfect love is what Christ did for you and for all lost mankind on His cross. It was there that He conquered the devil who had the power of the fear of death. "For this purpose the Son of God was manifested, that He might destroy the works of the devil," (1 John 3:8). Now is the time to demonstrate your trust in Jesus. Call upon Him to cleanse your soul by casting out the fear of death and any other fears that may be robbing you of His perfect peace. Because the love He has for you is perfect, He will do it! Just ask Him.

The Twenty-third Psalm is precious to believers all through life, but especially when life is ebbing away and you are about to be removed from loved ones. King David, who wrote this beloved Psalm, testifies so eloquently with these familiar words: "Yea, though I walk through the valley of the shadow of death, I will fear no evil; for You are with me." What could be more comforting, reassuring and faith building for you than this treasured portion of scripture?

> If you're not completely free from the fear of your death, reach out to Jesus.

What is it really like for a Christian to die? Scripture gives a picture of death being like walking through a valley with many shadows, including the shadowy fear of death. Be confident that this is not a lonely walk! The Creator of the Heavens, the earth, and all they contain will be walking with you, side by side, hand in hand. Dying brings God's children face to face with death, and immediately following, face to face with Jesus. Yes, dying is just like King David said. It is a walk with the Good Shepherd *through* death and fearing *no* evil, including the fear of death.

There are many who testify to experiencing supernatural life-after-death encounters. References are often made to walking through darkness while seeing "light at the end of the tunnel." Without questioning or judging the validity of these testimonials, we as Christians can know with absolute certainty that the light emerging out of darkness and dispelling it is no other light than the Light of Life which is Jesus!

Prayer:

Dear Jesus, how can I say thanks for Your perfect love given to me in countless ways? Help me to grow by Your grace to love You more. I know and believe that on Your cross, You destroyed the works of the enemy who was seeking to destroy me through my temptations, trials, and troubles. I humbly ask You to deliver me completely from the fear of death as promised in Your Word. Thank You for Your gracious shepherding care for me. Please continue to prepare me and my loved ones for my peaceful departure to be with You in all Your glory in Heaven above. I ask these things in Your Mighty Name. Amen.

I FEAR NO FOE,
WITH THEE AT HAND
TO BLESS;
ILLS HAVE NO WEIGHT,
AND TEARS NO BITTERNESS.
WHERE IS DEATH'S STING?
WHERE GRAVE THY
VICTORY?
I TRIUMPH STILL, IF THOU
ABIDE WITH ME!

— **William H. Monk** —
From: *Abide With Me*
Stanza 4, Public Domain

17

PASS AWAY
– FLY AWAY –
DEPARTURE

Scripture:

As he was praying, the appearance of his face changed, and his clothes became as bright as a flash of lightning. Two men, Moses and Elijah, appeared in glorious splendor, talking with Jesus. They spoke about *his departure*, which he was about to bring to fulfillment at Jerusalem.

Luke 9:29-31 NIV
[Emphasis added]

For me, to live is Christ, and to die is gain. But if I live on in the flesh, this will mean fruit from my labor; yet what I shall choose I cannot tell. For I am hard-pressed between the two, *having a desire to depart* and be with Christ, which is far better. Nevertheless, to remain in the flesh is more needful for you.

Philippians 1:21-24
[Emphasis added]

For I am already being poured out as a drink offering, and the time of *my departure* is at hand.

2 Timothy 4:6
[Emphasis added]

The days of our lives are seventy years; and if by reason of strength they are eighty years, yet their boast is only labor and sorrow; for it is soon cut off, and *we fly away.*

Psalm 90:10
[Emphasis added]

Meditation:

No doubt you wonder what actually is going to happen to you immediately following your last breath. There are many who believe that any answer to such a question is purely speculative. They say, "You cannot really know until you die; and maybe even then you will no longer have the capacity to know anything." Some Christians believe that when your body dies, your soul is consigned to a sort of "spiritual soul sleep" and on the day of the resurrection your spirit will be instantly awakened and be simultaneously joined to your new body. I will clearly show how false this teaching is. Take heart, dear friend!

Admittedly, scripture leaves some questions about life hereafter unanswered, or only gives symbolic pictures. And yet, the Bible has much clear and direct revelation about what actually does transpire upon the demise of the physical body. Jesus said, "And you shall know the truth, and the truth shall make you free" (John 8:32).

Regarding the question at hand, the four scripture passages quoted above declare the truth about what happens at death. Three phrases summarize what God's Word teaches on this subject: pass away, fly away, and departure. Essentially, all three expressions mean the same thing; namely, that at the moment of death the human spirit is immediately released to "pass away", to "fly away" and to "depart." James in his epistle proclaims the same truth. "For as the body without the spirit is dead, so faith without works is dead also" (James 2:26). Luke's account of Jesus being transfigured on the mountain relates how both Moses and Elijah, two great patriarchs of the Old Testament representing the Law and the Prophets, were very much alive in their spirit. And, in the spirit, they spoke of Jesus' *departure*, which He was to accomplish at Jerusalem. That conversation focused on the manner of Jesus' death by crucifixion, referring to it unmistakably as a *departure*. Jesus affirmed that His death on the cross would lead directly to His departure in the spirit. Listen to the last of His seven sayings while on the cross: "Father, into Your hands I commit My spirit" (Luke 23:46).

In addition, we have clear and amazing revelation from Paul's testimony as to what he believed and taught regarding the separation of the spirit from the body precisely when the body expires. His words are plain and to the point: "For the time of my departure is at hand" (2 Timothy 4:6). Again,

"For me to live is Christ, and to die is gain" (Philippians 1:21). What kind of "gain"? When will he possess it? Answer: immediately following the death of his body he would gain departure to go and be with the Lord, which is far better. What amazing grace the Lord offered Paul. He was actually given the choice: "Do you want to come home and be together with Me now, or would you prefer to continue your labors for Me and the saints" (Philippians 1:22-25). [Paraphrased] Paul's own words were; "Yet what I shall choose I cannot tell. For I am hard-pressed between the two" (Philippians 1:23a). Very few believers, if any, are given that choice. Yet we are promised the better of the two options as soon as God assists us to accomplish our departure just as He did for His Son Jesus, agonizing for our salvation on His cross!

A brief commentary on the Psalm 90 passage quoted above will conclude our Biblical inquiry about experiencing death as departure. Here we are told that the "normal" longevity of humans is seventy years. Yet, some are granted an additional ten years, but only by the strength that God gives. For sure these advancing years will not be without "labor and sorrow." Very likely you would say "amen" to this statement if you have lived to be eighty years or beyond.

Here is the good news God desires to speak to you in this passage. No matter how long you have lived as a believer trusting in Jesus, your death, whenever it comes, is a passing away from this life and an entrance into new life in Heaven with the Lord together with His angels and saints of all the ages.

And so dear friend, are you ready to pass away, to depart, to fly away and be with Jesus? It must be declared that the fate of those who have rejected personal faith in Jesus, refusing to believe on His Name and call upon Him for salvation, have a totally opposite destination after their death. Their spirit, which also separates from their deceased body, immediately descends to the place called "Hades" which defined by scripture means "the abode of the dead." Those who may believe that such a place does not exist need to consult Jesus! He spent the better part of three days in that "prison" proclaiming His total victory over death and the devil to those captive spirits who rejected the warning of impending judgment preached by Noah (1 Peter 3:18-20).

I readily acknowledge that this topic has led us into some pretty deep theological waters. But I trust that the Holy Spirit is revealing to you these truths and thus enabling you to experience the freedom He has prepared to give you. This will lead you to be fully prepared and ready to depart and, in your spirit, "fly away" to be with Him. Be fully assured that Jesus is eagerly awaiting your final and ultimate homecoming!

Prayer:

I bless You, Lord God, for the glorious truth of Your Word set forth in this meditation. Thank You, Holy Spirit, for burning away the fog of misconceptions and deceptions of false teachings regarding the separation of my spirit and my body when I die. Jesus, I thank You for helping me to believe that to die is great gain. Help me to joyfully anticipate my departure from this life and from my failing body to be with You in Heaven. In Your mercy and by Your grace, may it be soon. I pray in Your holy Name. Amen.

I AM RESOLVED NO
LONGER TO LINGER,
CHARMED
BY THE WORLD'S DELIGHT;
THINGS THAT ARE
HIGHER, THINGS THAT ARE
NOBLER, THESE HAVE
ALLURED MY SIGHT.

— **James H. Fillmore** —

From: I Am Resolved
Living Hymns, pg. 517

18

SETTING YOUR HOUSE IN ORDER

LEGAL MEASURES

Scripture:

In those days Hezekiah was sick and near death. And Isaiah the prophet, the son of Amoz, went to him and said to him, "Thus says the Lord: 'Set your house in order, for you shall die and not live' ".

Isaiah 38:1

Now there stood by the cross of Jesus His mother, and His mother's sister, Mary the wife of Clopas, and Mary Magdalene. When Jesus therefore saw His mother, and the disciple whom He loved standing by, He said to His mother, "Woman, behold your son!" Then He said to the disciple, "Behold your mother!" And from that hour that disciple took her to his own home.

John 19:25-27

Meditation:

Life is unpredictable. As the saying goes, "You never know what a day may bring." Accordingly, wise and prudent adults whether married, single, a widow or a widower, will consult an attorney and draw up legal papers specifying the terms of their will, and the distribution of their estate.

However, some individuals procrastinate and fail to perform this task. It is not too late to make these legal arrangements even after the much-dreaded words are spoken by your physician: "I regret to inform you that it is now time to set your house in order. Your physical condition indicates that you are not likely to recover." King Hezekiah received that same sobering diagnosis from the Lord delivered by His prophet Isaiah.

It is interesting to note that even in Bible times; various cultures specified certain organizational tasks to be performed by those who became terminally ill. Another classic example of this practice was carried out by Jesus just prior to the time of His death. Most likely, His stepfather Joseph was deceased at the time of His crucifixion. This circumstance would have necessitated Jesus' responsibility, being the firstborn son, to make arrangements for the care of His mother. Many widows were completely cut off from any means of support. This indicates how loving and compassionate it was of Jesus to adequately care for His mother's future needs. Accordingly, He chose John the apostle He loved so much, and directed him to "adopt" His mother Mary into his own household.

All previous meditations have focused exclusively on spiritual matters dealing with the Scriptural exhortations to *Prepare to Meet Your God*. This message is different. It deals with practical temporal choices and tasks, which are also important.

If you have not yet drawn up your last will and testament, it is not too late. Nor is it a complicated procedure. A phone call to an attorney is all it takes to begin this task. A lawyer will gladly explain the process of drafting a will in language you will understand. If this task seems unpleasant, awkward, or too expensive, bear in mind that if you die *in testate* [having no valid will], the court system has full authority to impose a distribution of your assets, as they deem appropriate. This legal ruling does not currently apply to all States. Also, there are numerous legal statutes from State to State and court to court which govern the distribution of your estate even though you *have* established your will. Examples would be multiple marriages subsequent to divorce, the eligibility of children from these unions as potential heirs, and the legal interpretation of the specifications of your will based on these and other provisos.

Should you be a widow or a widower, a second necessity to address in setting your house in order would be to go through the proper legal channels for appointing a guardian for any of your children who are minors at the time of your passing.

Thirdly, you may want to decide whether to donate one or more of your vital organs and/or specific body tissues for possible transplant purposes or other medical procedures. Such preferences need to be stated in writing, comprising a document known as a "Power of Attorney for Health Care." The person you select may be an attorney, but other family or persons of legal age are eligible and may be appointed to serve. You should select a person knowledgeable about your wishes, values, and religious beliefs, in whom you have trust and confidence, and who knows how you feel about health care.

Additional provisions may be included in the same document, which pertain to medical treatment procedures if, and when, your physical condition becomes serious enough to mandate consideration of extraordinary measures.

Common examples include the surgical insertion of a feeding tube when normal intake capacities are no longer viable. Another might be the dire need to use a ventilator when a patient is no longer able to sustain life by normal breathing. You might also want to specify restrictions prohibiting resuscitative measures when death becomes apparent. Other extraordinary treatments may apply according to the particular debilitating health problems of each individual patient.

Consult your physician or other health caregivers to provide the necessary forms, as well as skilled help to interpret and assist you in completing the documents. Since these weighty and complex decisions can be difficult, I recommend that due consideration be given to your desires *and* those of your surviving family.

Another category of set-your-house-in-order arrangements would be informing immediate family members of your directives as to how your earthly remains are to be treated. If you have already selected a particular mortuary and a representative mortician, he or she would be pleased to know prior to your passing whether your intent is to have your remains embalmed and buried in the traditional manner or cremated. A third, less common option, but still elected by some, is the donation of all remains for medical research purposes.

A final area of arrangements concerns stating preferences regarding your funeral or memorial service. Most likely, your spouse and/or family members will be respective of your requests and appreciate your assistance. If you have membership in a local church, your pastor will be eager to offer help with advance preparation for your funeral or memorial service. Should you have no affiliation with a local church, most funeral homes have chapel facilities.

The director of the home would be pleased to request the services of a clergyperson representing your denominational preference to work with you and your loved ones in planning your service. You may have one or more scripture passages you would like to have read. You may also choose one or more hymns or gospel songs which you believe would bring special inspiration and comfort to your loved ones and friends attending the service. Lastly, if you have served your country in active duty in one of the branches of the armed forces, you may request military honors be a part of the graveside service.

In your individual case, there may be other important and helpful tasks necessary to complete while setting your house in order. Be open to suggestions from family members. Doing so could ease their burden of making numerous difficult decisions in the emotionally painful time of grief and sorrow.

Prayer:

Dear God: Thank You for revealing to me through Your Word that setting my house in order is important to You, as well as to me and my loved ones. I ask for Your wisdom and strength to complete these tasks in a manner pleasing to You and helpful to my survivors. Thank You for the promise of Your peace attending all the necessary arrangements for a godly closure to my earthly pilgrimage. In the Name of Your Holy Son, Jesus, I pray. Amen.

19

ANGELIC ESCORT ON YOUR TRIP TO HEAVEN

Scripture:

For He shall give His angels charge over you, to keep you in all your ways.

Psalm 91:11

The angel of the Lord encamps all around those who fear Him and delivers them.

Psalm 34:7

There was a certain rich man who was clothed in purple and fine linen and fared sumptuously every day. But there was a certain beggar named Lazarus, full of sores, who was laid at his gate, desiring to be fed with the crumbs which fell from the rich man's table. Moreover the dogs came and licked his sores. So it was that the beggar died, and was carried by the angels to Abraham's bosom. The rich man also died and was buried.

Luke 16:19-22

Meditation:

Have you ever heard the saying, "God is good" followed by this reply, "All the time"? These brief affirmative confessions are based on what the Bible states in Psalm 23:6 "Surely goodness and mercy shall follow me all the days of my life; and I will dwell in the house of the Lord forever." Dear friend, can you say in retrospect that this testimony of King David's life is also true of your experience? If so, I want to assure you that God's goodness and mercy will continue to attend you no less during these very difficult remaining days of your life on earth!

God's goodness is expressed toward us in more numerous ways and situations than we can comprehend with our finite minds. This meditation will focus on one particular expression of God's goodness that I will call "supernatural providential care through the various ministries of angels."

As you read the scriptures about angels quoted above, were you somewhat surprised to learn that Jesus has assigned at least two of His angels, (and more if needed), as your very own "secret service agents"? Their assignment is to protect and guard you *in all your ways* and for *all your days*! How good of God to do that. There is much more of His goodness channeled exclusively through angels. Read on.

During these current days of global terrorism, virtually everyone is concerned about security—international security, homeland security, and personal security. Rest assured, God is concerned about our security more than any of us are! How do we know that? Because He has told us so in His Word. "The angel of the Lord encamps all around those who fear Him and delivers them" (Psalm 34:7). Can you picture this? A single angel is all that is needed to keep you [or a large company of persons] totally secure day and night! This ministering spirit utilizes a strategy analogous to the 360-degree sweep of radar surveillance continuously monitoring for potential threats from enemy combatants. This analogy is based upon the phrase "encamps all around" in Psalm 34:7 quoted above. During the westward movement of the pioneers in America, they frequently encamped by parking their covered wagons in a full circle so as to have better protection from wild animals and hostile Indians.

I have developed this particular facet of super-natural angelic care to build up your faith and enable you to be free from anxiety about your loved ones after you are gone. Just believe His promise that His angels will guard and keep them in all their ways for all their days. Be confident that you can entrust them to God's goodness and mercy as you speak your final farewell to them.

Now let us focus on the final ministry of *your* angels, which will commence the instant your body expires. Fasten your "spiritual seatbelt"! You may be "wowed" as you grasp the truth that Jesus, who is the Lord of hosts (all angels), will dispatch two or more angels to escort you to your eternal destiny. Admittedly, this revelation is awesomely supernatu-ral, and highly mystical. Yet, it is entirely true! It's going to happen. It's going to happen to you! God alone knows the day and the hour.

Here is the revelation I'm referring to: "So it was that the beggar died, and was carried by the angels to Abraham's bosom" (Luke 16:22). "Abraham's bosom" was a Biblical phrase for God's abode in Heaven. Dear friend, be fully persuaded that Jesus, was not speaking hypothetically, figuratively, symbolically or allegorically. He was talking straight talk about two specific individuals who were very likely His contemporaries. This we know because of His reference to a *certain* rich man whom He chose to keep anonymous. Next, He made reference to a *certain* beggar whose name was Lazarus. These two persons lived in history and, in the end, experienced a very real fate. One was destined to Heaven and the other was destined to Hell. Heaven is a real place. No less, Hell is a real place.

You will recall from a previous meditation that God's Word declares upon death of the physical body, the spirits of believers in Jesus, and the spirits of unbelievers as well, are immediately separated from the body. At precisely that instant, believers trusting Jesus alone for their eternal salvation will be granted an angelic escort all the way to the presence of the Father in Heaven. How long will the journey take? That remains part of the mystery. Why does your spirit need to be *carried* by angels? Here is my answer. Our Father God has prearranged for you to be escorted by angels because it will be a supernatural "ride" through supernatural realms to a supernatural place you have not previously visited! Personally, I believe that our spirit, though free from the body, would still be very much foreign to the celestial realms. Therefore, a "solo flight" through space and infinitely beyond would require a "navigational skill" that any freshly "airborne" human spirit would not likely possess. Forgive me for trying to explain the inexplicably mysterious. Even so, I hope you will join me in the excitement of surmising a bit about the *reality* of these truths and in offering an interpretation that excludes even a hint of them being mythical fantasies!

Billy Graham's book, *Angels: God's Secret Agents* contains an eight-page section called "Christians at Death." The following excerpt speaks profoundly about our future angelic escort to Heaven.

> In another connection I have already mentioned Lazarus, whom angels escorted to Abraham in Heaven. This story has always been a tremendous comfort to me as I think about death. I will actually be taken by angels into the presence of God. These ministering spirits who have helped me here

so often will be with me in my last great battle on earth. Death is a battle, a profound crisis event. Paul calls it "the last enemy," (1 Corinthians 15:26). While the sting of death has been removed by the work of Christ on the cross, and by His resurrection, yet the crossing of this valley still stimulates fear and mystery. However, angels will be there to help us. [1]

Prayer:

Dear Jesus: Thank You for revealing to me that You are the Lord of hosts with myriads of angels at Your command. How blessed I have been through-out my life to be guarded and kept in all my ways by specific angels You gave charge over me. Lord, I am so grateful to You for the joyous and peaceful assurance I have in knowing that angels will one day be escorting me to the eternal habitation you have prepared. I ask You to keep me focused on this glorious expectation. Thank You for Your grace, which day by day is leading me victoriously through my battle of sickness unto death. In Your mighty Name I pray. Amen.

[1] Billy Graham, *Angels: God's Secret Agents*, (Doubleday & Company Inc., Garden City, NY, 1975).

BUT GOD WILL
REDEEM MY SOUL
FROM THE POWER
OF THE GRAVE,
FOR HE SHALL
RECEIVE ME.

Psalm 49:15

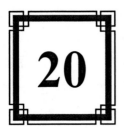

20

SEEING THE INVISIBLE

Scripture:

For our light affliction, which is but for a moment, is working for us a far more exceeding and eternal weight of glory, while we do not look at the things which are seen, but at the things which are not seen. For the things which are seen are temporary, but the things which are not seen are eternal.

2 Corinthians 4:17-18

Meditation:

To say that Christians are

those who "look at the things which are not seen" is to declare that they can "see the invisible." That sounds like a direct contradiction, but not when the statement is properly understood. When Paul uses the terms "light affliction" and "but for a moment," he is contrasting the circumstances of earthly afflictions with the "eternal weight of glory." This entirely new perspective and the glorious appearances, which will accompany it, will be revealed immediately following death and your spirit's transport to Heaven itself. Moreover, the sufferings and afflictions, which ultimately lead to the death of this temporal body actually have a redemptive purpose. This is indicated by Paul's phrase "*working for us* an exceeding and eternal weight of glory."

A significant part of accepting our mortality is to honestly admit that the things, which are seen, are temporary. This temporal earthly existence with all of its beauty, pleasures, and joys, combined with the dark side of disease, pain, death, and separation is sending us a message loud and clear: we are not to consider ourselves at home in this earthly life. During our time spent here, we are strangers, foreigners, pilgrims, and aliens.

Our ultimate destiny can never be reached here. As creatures made by God in His own image, we are designed to *transcend* this earthly habitation! The Bible says it this way: "Also He has put eternity in their hearts, except that no one can find out the work that God does from the beginning to the end" (Ecclesiastes 3:11). Elsewhere we read: "For here we have no continuing city, but we seek the one to come" (Hebrews 13:14).

> Afflictions, which lead to death, have a redemptive purpose.

Dear friend, as you have journeyed thus far through the goals and the tasks of *Prepare to Meet Your God,* you know that there are struggles involved in this venture. Just as you are struggling to endure the pain resulting from the deterioration of body functions, there is also the struggle of resigning, relinquishing, and letting go of all that is near and dear to you in this life. Making this transition from the temporal to the eternal requires a measure of faith and trust in God that perhaps seems beyond your ability just now. But take heart! Jesus lovingly beckons you to come to Him and believe in Him.

This is His gracious summons, which will enable you to look to Him. He is the sum and the substance of all things that are eternal. Be blessed right now, as you learn from Jesus how powerfully He will execute your transition from the earthly to the eternal. "Let not your heart be troubled; you believe in God, believe also in Me. In My Father's house are many mansions; if it were not so, I would have told you. I go to prepare a place for you. And if I go and prepare a place for you, I will come again and receive you to Myself; that where I am, there you may be also" (John 14:1-3).

While hanging on the cross, with only moments of life remaining, Jesus cried out with a victory shout exclaiming, *"It is finished!"* Thus He proclaimed that His earthly mission was perfectly completed, fully accomplished! By sacrificing His holy body and His sinless life, He slammed shut the doors of Hell and opened wide the gates of Heaven for all who truly believe and trust in Him. As your great High Priest seated at the right hand of His Father, Jesus prays for you. In so doing, He is shutting down the gravitational pull of this earthly life on your soul. The result is a new gravity beginning to set in. Compare it to a spacecraft on its way to the moon. Gradually, earth's gravity loses its drag as the tugging force of the moon's gravity begins to take over. Are you beginning to experience Heaven's gravitational tug and pull? By God's grace, you will!

As the curtain of this life begins to lower, God is tenderly calling you to focus more keenly on your heavenly destiny. His design is to train your eyes by means of His gift of faith to *see the invisible*. In this context, how appropriate are the lyrics of this chorus: "Turn your eyes upon Jesus, look full in His wonderful face; and the things of earth will grow strangely dim in the light of His glory and grace."[1] As you know, there will be no "hold" placed on the steady countdown of your remaining days. Your capacity to "hang on" will gradually slip away. Have no fear. Rather, be confident that Jesus, your Good Shepherd, will not allow you to slip out of the grip of His strong hands and loving arms! He, who opened the eyes of those born blind, will open your spiritual eyes and enable you to see with 20/20 vision the vistas of His glorious inheritance prepared for you in Heaven above.

This meditation will conclude with the story of Saint Stephen, the first Christian martyr. He was stoned to death because of his testimony of proclaiming Jesus to be the Messiah. "But he, being full of the Holy Spirit, gazed into Heaven and saw the glory of God, and Jesus standing at the right hand of God, and said, 'Look! I see the Heavens opened and the Son of Man standing at the right hand of God' " (Acts 7:55-56).

Most likely, you are not dying as a martyr. Nonetheless, you are having to endure the compounded affliction of mounting physical pain, emotional trauma, and the stressful anguish of being severed from your dearest loved ones. Allow me to state it one more time. As the Apostle Paul described this very experience, he dared to use language that borders on being insulting. He said, "This affliction is *light* and will last *but for a moment*." He uses these two figures of speech ("light" and "moment") to draw a stark contrast with the "far more exceeding and eternal weight of glory." Indeed! The grand and glorious transition from this world to the entrance of Heaven itself is that radical, that transforming, and that awesome!

Prayer:

Dear heavenly Father: I thank You for all the grace You have promised which is bringing my life to a good and godly closure. Please forgive me for all the times I have been earthbound and not mindful of Your holy summons to look not to the things that are temporal and transient, but to the things, which are unseen and eternal. I truly need You to open my eyes and fix my gaze upon Jesus and the destiny of Heaven He is preparing for me. How great to know that Your strength will enable me to endure all the afflictions of my latter days and make them redemptive as You usher me into Your eternal glory. Jesus, I surrender all to You. Take me and lead me home. In Your precious Name I pray. Amen.

[1] Helen Howarth Lemmel, "Turn your eyes upon Jesus," 1922, Public domain.

IN THE MULTITUDE
OF MY ANXIETIES
WITHIN ME
YOUR COMFORTS
DELIGHT MY SOUL

Psalm 94:19

21

HAVING THE RIGHT KIND OF ANXIETY

Scripture:

For we know that if the earthly tent we live in is destroyed, we have a building from God, a house not made with hands, eternal in the Heavens. Here indeed we groan, and long to put on our heavenly dwelling, so that by putting it on we may not be found naked. For while we are still in this tent, we sigh with anxiety; not that we would be unclothed, but that we would be further clothed, so that what is mortal may be swallowed up by life. He who has prepared us for this very thing is God, who has given us the Spirit as a guarantee.

2 Corinthians 5:1-5 RSV

Meditation:

You are invited to "listen in" to the instructions the Apostle Paul gave the church in the city of Corinth regarding issues relating to severe illness, which may or may not lead to death. First, there should be no anxiety about being "un-clothed" (becoming a naked spirit without a body). These verses from God's Word are loaded with metaphors and symbolic language. How else could Paul hope to explain the inexplicable or describe the indescribable, or communicate the infinite realties of eternity in mere human terms? Making and selling tents supported his apostolic ministry. What a fitting metaphor to describe the frailty and limited endur-ance of our physical body—an earthly tent! Canvas tents are subject to becoming tattered and torn. So too, our physical bodies will eventually be destroyed in one-way or another.

How quickly and dramatically the metaphor shifts to a "house not made with hands, eternal in the Heavens." This is not just any house, but a specially prepared house designed and made by none other than God Himself! Paul's use of the term "house" does not refer to a piece of celestial real estate, which you will call "home" when you get to Heaven. This house "eternal in the Heavens" refers to an entirely new resurrection body with which God will clothe all believers who are already pre-registered citizens of Heaven. This body will never age, become diseased, and be subject to injuries, become afflicted and weak, nor for any other reason be destroyed! That's why it is called a body, which will be *eternal* in the Heavens!

God's Word continues to inform believers how to be gripped by this awesome promise, which awaits us. Paul is saying that groaning pains caused by a grave illness are better endured by sighing aspirations and deep longing to put on our heavenly dwelling. Reflect for a few moments upon God's "clothing" prepared and given to us while on earth. Jesus said, "Consider the lilies of the field, how they grow: they neither toil nor spin; and yet I say to you that even Solomon in all his glory was not arrayed like one of these... Will He not much more clothe you, O you of little faith" (Matthew 6:28-30)?

Our Creator God's first clothing gift was our physical body. Life as we know it in our "earthly tent" is beautiful because we are created in His image, and "in Him we live, and move and have our being" (Acts 17:28). Furthermore, Christ has clothed our spirit and soul with His perfect right-eousness. This occurs as He gradually imparts to us the garments of His very own character virtues.

> How can you be assured that you are included in the company of believing saints?

Finally, God will consummate our becoming an entirely new creation in Christ by clothing our spirit with a perfect resurrection body fashioned like His glorious Resurrection Body. This is how the promise reads in scripture: "For our citizenship is in Heaven, from which we also eagerly wait for the Savior, the Lord Jesus Christ, who will transform our lowly body that it may be con-formed to His glorious body, according to the work-ing by which He is able even to subdue all things to Himself" (Philippians 3:20-21).

Let's talk about the wrong and the right kind of anxiety, which is appropriate for believers drawing near to life's end. Paul said, "While we are still in this earthly tent, we sigh with anxiety." This anxiety, for the Christian, is *not* based on the process of physical dying. Paul describes this event as being "unclothed" (becoming a naked spirit without a body). Here is another way of stating this truth. Upon expiring, our spirit is released from the "destroyed tent" and is not yet clothed with the new body, which body awaits us on the day of our resurrection. This is the all-important truth: The Lord earnestly desires that we remain totally free from all anxiety about death itself and about being a spirit without a body until Christ returns to earth at the end of the age! I fully trust that as you read the scriptures together with the meditations, and pray the prayers of this book, your spirit will be *renewed daily*.

What then, is the right kind of anxiety referred to in the phrase "being further clothed"? Speaking of God's gift of a resurrection body fashioned after Christ's glorious resurrection body, Paul says we should indeed be anxiously awaiting to receive this divine clothing! As death draws near, surely we should be eager, hopeful, and yes, truly anxious to be clothed with *immortality* as God has promised in His Word: "So when this corruptible has put on incorruption, and this *mortal has put on immortality,* then shall be brought to pass the saying that is written: *"Death is swallowed up in victory, O Death, where is your sting? O Hades, where is your victory"* (1 Corinthians 15:54-55). Moreover, this God-ordained form of anxiety should characterize every Christian's life, not just those drawing close to death's door!

There is yet another metaphor to be considered. When the Lord God gives the "signal", Jesus, accompanied by His angels, will return to earth. What happens next? It will be what one Negro spiritual song describes as *"Dat Great Gittin' Up Mornin".* The Bible declares that on that great day, "What is mortal may be swallowed up by life. He who has prepared us for this very thing is God, who has given us the Spirit as a guarantee" (2 Corinthians 5:4b-5 RSV). The resurrection power and life of Jesus will make it happen. Quickly!

How can you be fully assured that you are included in this glorious company of believing saints destined to be delivered from mortality to immortality? God gives us complete assurance by giving us His Holy Spirit as a guarantee. Everyone who truly believes in Jesus, having personally received Him as his or her own Savior and Lord, has also received the precious gift of the Holy Spirit. Yes, the *person* of the Holy Spirit lives within you. He actually dwells in your body, making it the temple of His holy presence! Since it was this same Holy Spirit who raised Jesus from the dead and clothed Him with His resurrection body, all Christians have received the "guarantee" of their own bodily resurrection to be accomplished by the person of the Holy Spirit. There is more! The Holy Spirit whom Jesus promised would "be with you forever" will also inhabit your perfect resurrection body for all eternity. Doesn't this call for a holy anxiety, a joyous expectation for God to fulfill all that He has guaranteed?!

Dear friend, I trust that you have now been enabled to release all fearful anxiety about the remaining time you have to dwell in your earthly body. I pray this meditation has freed you to have a good and godly anxiety about being clothed with a glorious resurrection body fashioned like Jesus' body! He is speaking to you now. He makes a tremendous claim and follows it with a very penetrating question. Jesus said, "I am the resurrection and the life. He who believes in Me, though he may die; yet he shall live. And whoever lives and believes in Me shall never die. Do you believe this" (John 11:25-26).

Prayer:

Father God, I am so amazed and so thankful for this revelation from Your Word. You have said, "Have no anxiety about anything." I confess that I have been anxious about my illness and facing death. Please breathe Your peace into my soul and drive out all my negative thoughts and emotions. By Your Holy Spirit's power, enable me to be anxious and eager to be clothed with a new resurrection body, like the glorious body of Your Son. I desperately need your gifts of faith, hope and love which will help me to bear all things, believe all things, hope all things, and endure all things. Holy Father, in Your great mercy, please hear my prayer offered in Jesus' Name. Amen.

22

ACHIEVING AN ATTITUDE OF RELINQUISH-MENT

Scripture:

For none of us lives to himself, and no one dies to himself. For if we live, we live to the Lord, and if we die, we die to the Lord. Therefore, whether we live or die, we are the Lord's. For to this end Christ died and rose and lived again, that He might be Lord of both the dead and the living.

Romans 14:7-9

Meditation:

Dear friend, you may be aware that many people upon receiving the "official notice" of their impending death are not mentally or emotionally capable of hearing or accepting such dreaded news. Therefore, the immediate response is frequently characterized by being stunned, shocked, angered, and overwhelmed. This rush of negative emotions commonly leads to a subsequent negative frame of mind expressed as denial and depression. I am probably not telling you anything new because you have been experiencing, to one degree or another, some of these same thoughts and emotions.

It is my sincere hope that by reading this book, and praying the prayers, you are experiencing much love and comfort from the Lord and will be lifted up from any despair and hopelessness. By God's grace, you will no longer need to resort to denial as a way to cope. The Lord is preparing you to stare death in the face and fight the good fight of faith with His divine help. Realizing that you still have dignity, worth, purpose, and destiny will help you to be victorious in this struggle. If these positive affirmations about your personhood are only perceived dimly in your own eyes, rest assured that in God's eyes, you continue to be esteemed very highly!

For your immediate family and loved ones, working through their sorrow and grief begins in earnest after you have passed away. For some, this is a lengthy process. But for you, working through your sorrow and grief is compressed into a relatively brief period of time making it intense and difficult. However, Jesus is working with you and all your dear loved ones in your sorrowing and grieving. Surely you can identify with the sentiments of this scripture: "Is it nothing to you, all you who pass by? Behold and see if there is any sorrow like my sorrow" (Lamentations 1:12a). Be comforted by these words also: "He was despised and rejected by men, a Man of sorrows and acquainted with grief. And we hid, as it were, our faces from Him" (Isaiah 53:3).

> Your departure is a divine appointment, God is summoning you.

Take courage knowing that Jesus has experienced grief and sorrow, which far surpasses that of any living person. Therefore, He is able to fully identify, sympathize, and empathize with you by actually entering into the brokenness of your heart with His healing balm. This in part is the meaning of the saying, "For none of us lives to himself, and no one dies to himself. For if we live, we live to the Lord; and if we die, we die to the Lord" (Romans 14:7-8).

The design of this book has been to take you through various critically important steps necessary to be prepared to meet your God. Admittedly, this process is proving to be a somewhat painful and difficult experience. The specific goal of this meditation is to assist you in achieving an attitude of relinquishment.

The dictionary gives a list of synonyms for relinquishment. Some of them are to yield, to resign, to surrender, to concede, to abandon, and to waive. The initial step is to know to whom your relinquishment is to be expressed. Clearly, the answer is Christ, who indeed continues to be your Lord during the remainder of your living, your dying, and after you depart from this life. For believers in Christ, dying is never an isolated, strictly individualistic event. Your passing will affect many persons deeply, even as your living has done for years. But most importantly, your dying will *be to the Lord!* For this reason, it is to Jesus, your Master and your Lord, that you are to humbly relinquish your life, all those persons whom you dearly love, and all the earthly possessions which you highly prize.

Remember that your departure is a divine appointment with God. He is sovereignly summoning you by saying, "It is time now to let go, to yield, to release everyone and everything. Now is the time for you to come home and dwell with Me." To answer this call requires *relinquishment*. It is nothing less than a submissive attitude of agreement, an act of obedience, and a consummate step, which prepares you to "die unto the Lord." Doing so should not be considered so much a duty but rather a blessed *delight*. Christ's very last words from the cross, spoken just prior to His final breath, dramatically define both the attitude and the act of relinquishment. "Father, into Your Hands, I commit My spirit" (Luke 23:46).

I sincerely hope you will be inspired by the experience of two individuals whose dire sickness drove them to pray powerful prayers of relinquishment, which prayers set them free. Catherine Marshall, in her book A *Man Called Peter,* tells the story of a missionary who had served the Lord faithfully for several years when suddenly she was stricken by a disease, which resulted in her being bedridden for eight years. Of this woman Marshall writes:

> During those long years, she had steadily and persistently asked God "Why?" She could not understand why she should be laid on the shelf when she was doing the Lord's work. There was rebellion in her heart, and the drums of mutiny rolled every now and then. The burden of her prayers was that God should make her well, in order that she might return to the mission field. But nothing happened. Finally, worn out with failure of these prayers and with a desperate sort of resignation within her, she prayed, 'All right Lord, I give in. If I am to be sick for the rest of my life, I bow to Thy will. I want Thee even more than I want health. It is for Thee to decide.' [1]

Immediately following this story, Mrs. Marshall continues by sharing her own experience of being suddenly attacked by a disease, which eventually drove her to praying a prayer of relinquishment. Her testimony follows:

> Suddenly, an inner illumination, playing on the missionary's experience, revealed to me my mistakes in prayer. I had been demanding

of God. I had claimed health as my right. Furthermore, I had not faced reality. The right way, then, must be the only way left—that of submission and surrender to the situation as it was. Privately, with tears eloquent of the reality of what I was doing, I lay in bed and prayed, 'Lord, I've done everything I've known how to do, and it hasn't been good enough. I'm desperately weary of the struggle of trying to persuade You to give me what I want. I'm beaten, whipped, through. If You want me to be an invalid for the rest of my life, all right. Here I am. Do anything You like with me and my life.'[2]

I rejoice to tell you that God miraculously healed both of these women! They were set free! However, be assured that my intention is not to present these illustrations of praying the prayer of relinquishment as some sort of a "formula" which will motivate God to miraculously heal *all* the sick, including those who are sick unto death. The Bible declares that God "does whatever He pleases" (Psalm 115:3). We are not at liberty to program Him or to try to fit Him into the "box" of our personal will. However, His Word teaches that the physical death of a believer's body is, in reality, the ultimate healing! Physical pain, diseases, and old-age infirmities are terminated forever. That in itself is a miracle, the results of which last eternally. I consider this ultimate healing to be another dimension of the deep meaning of "dying unto the Lord."

Guidelines for your own prayer:

I sincerely trust that the Holy Spirit will enable you either silently or audibly, from the inner depths of your heart and mind, to pray your own personal prayer of relinquishment. In doing so, you will be offering to God an "amen" to His Word presented in this meditation. The Lord bless and keep you.

[1] Catherine Marshal, *A Man Called Peter (New York, NY, McGraw-Hill, 1951)*, 177-178 Copyright transferred to Baker Publishing Group, Grand Rapids, MI – Used by permission.
[2] *Ibid.*

23

WHAT GOD IS PREPARING FOR YOU PART I

Scripture:

Let not your heart be troubled; you believe in God, believe also in Me. In My Father's house are many mansions; if it were not so, I would have told you. I go to prepare a place for you. And if I go and prepare a place for you, I will come again and receive you to Myself; that where I am, there you may be also.

John 14:1-3

Meditation:

Many of the meditation topics in this book have been devoted to the all-important theme of preparing to meet your God. Let us turn this "coin" over and talk about what God is preparing for *you* in Heaven.

It has been said, "Heaven is a prepared place for a prepared people." That saying is partly based upon the teaching of Jesus quoted above. As Jesus was preparing His chosen apostles and believing disciples for His ascension back to His Father in Heaven, they were both confused and sorrowful. Jesus said to them, "A little while, and you will not see Me; and again a little while, and you will see Me, because I go to the Father." To which they replied, "What is this that He says to us, 'A little while'? We do not know what He is saying" (John 16:16, 18). The disciples were sorrowful. Jesus knew this when He counseled them saying, "Let not your heart be troubled."

Dear friend, as your time of departure draws near, undoubtedly you and your loved ones are sorrowful. For those who truly love each other, separation is always painful. The comforting counsel Jesus gave to His followers is the same counsel He gives to you and your loved ones. "Let not your heart be troubled." Receive His peace, which will quiet your heart and calm your spirit. His special mission on earth was to prepare you to be reconciled to your heavenly Father. Upon His return to Heaven, His special mission was to prepare a place *for you* among the many dwelling places in glory above. Jesus was not speaking about some wishful, fanciful, pious pie in the sky by-and-by. He spoke the real truth about your future in eternity. It's going to happen! He also said, with complete assurance, that if He would go away to prepare a place for you, He certainly would come back to bring you safely there. The comforting hope Jesus is declaring to you is that because you love Him and He loves you, you are destined to be together forever! Forever together! I trust that the perfect peace of your Savior is removing all confusion, trouble, and fear from your heart.

> In My Father's house are many mansions... I go to prepare a place for you.

He has more good news for you and your loved ones. When you gave your heart and your life to

Him, He instructed one of His angels to inscribe your name in His Book of Life. This means that you have become a pre-registered citizen of Heaven! As a citizen of Heaven you will, as it were, hold a "certified title" to a parcel of "celestial real estate." Believe this! There will be no mortgage because it is a gift, paid in full by Jesus! Is there a Bible verse to support that statement? Yes! "The Spirit bears witness with our spirit that we are children of God, and if children, then heirs—heirs of God and joint heirs with Christ" (Romans 8:16-17). In this earthly life, whatever material worth we inherit is a gift. How much more does the same truth apply to our inheritance from our Father God and His precious Son Jesus! Bear this in mind also: citizens of Heaven—God's Kingdom—will never pay any taxes, including inheritance tax!

There is still more good news. The place Jesus has gone to prepare for you is more than a dwelling place. He is also preparing for you a place of *service* in His everlasting Kingdom. How boring eternity would become if there was only idleness—sitting around, hanging around, lying around, and "floating" around plucking harps. For the children of God who have already gone home to glory, scripture tells us, "Therefore they are before the throne of

God, and *serve* Him day and night in His temple" (Revelation 7:15a). [Emphasis added]

Unfortunately, some people during their life on earth live much of their lives unfulfilled, devoid of meaning and lasting joy because they never really found *their place* in life. They are sometimes referred to as those who "missed their calling." This is often said regarding their careers, but it also applies in marriage, in family, and other interpersonal relationships.

Praise God, there will be no "misfits" in the Kingdom of Heaven! Quite the contrary, you can fully anticipate that God has uniquely designed and gifted you for the uniquely designated *place* where you will be joined and knitted together for service with the saints of all the ages! This is what the Bible refers to as your "divine destiny".

I sincerely believe that these truths are a significant part of the deeper meaning of Jesus' statement, "I go to prepare a *place* for you" (John 14:20). [Emphasis added] Let it also be said that as Jesus wisely places you in the spot He has prepared, you will always be joyfully and purposefully walking in the "good, acceptable, and perfect will of God" (Romans 12:2) and thoroughly enjoying every moment of it!

Prayer:

Lord Jesus, thank You so much for exciting my heart with all the awesome things You are preparing for me upon my soon arrival in Heaven. I bless You for Your wonderful truths and promises, which speak so, clearly about my eternal future and perfect place in Your Kingdom. I am so grateful for Your ministry to my troubled heart, and filling me with Your peace. What a foretaste of glory divine. I pray in Your holy Name. Amen.

24

WHAT GOD IS PREPARING FOR YOU PART II

Scripture:

But as it is written: "Eye has not seen, nor ear heard, nor have entered into the heart of man the things which God has prepared for those who love Him," But God has revealed them to us through His Spirit. For the Spirit searches all things; yes, the deep things of God.

1 Corinthians 2:9-10

For we are His workmanship, created in Christ Jesus for good works, which God prepared before-hand that we should walk in them.

Ephesians 2:10

Meditation:

The previous meditation revealed what God is preparing for you in Heaven in terms of your eternal *place* of dwelling. It also introduced the subject of what God is preparing for you by way of *serving* Him in His everlasting Kingdom. This meditation further develops this same topic. Both of the passages quoted above speak directly about what God has prepared in Heaven for those who love Him and who are called according to His purposes. So what is all this divine preparation about? In a single word— *work!* Not just any kind of work. These "good works" are designed exclusively for you according to your talents and gifts. In other words, you and your *servant tasks* will be perfectly matched! During this eternal service, always and forever, you will sense being wholly adequate, completely fulfilled, and thoroughly enthused. This is true because you are God's workmanship!

Dear friend, because this truth is so exciting and

important for you to grasp, I want to state it again. God is saying that you are a unique creation of His, with a unique personality, endowed with unique gifts and abilities for a unique ministry of service designed precisely with you in mind! That may sound like flattery, but it is the truth—God's truth, not mine! Please allow me to say it one more time in yet another way. Because you are God's work-manship created in Christ Jesus for good works which God prepared beforehand that we should walk in them" (Ephesians 2:10), the Kingdom of God both in Heaven and on earth *needs you!* You will be performing a highly significant role in God's eternal plan for the nations of the earth.

I trust that a sense of joyous expectation will well up within you as you begin to "see" what your eyes have never seen, and "hear" what your ears have never heard, and as God continues to plant sacred truths in your heart, which have never entered there before, a sense of joyous expectation will begin to well up within you. Above all else, this is what God desires for you as He prepares to launch you into His heavenly Kingdom!

In closing, I return to Paul's statement concerning the things God has prepared for those who love

Him. Note how at first he says that these things are *concealed* mysteries hidden away in God's private thoughts beyond the reach of our eyes, ears, and heart. And yet, ever so suddenly, the Holy Spirit is introduced as the One who *reveals* these things. What things? The things God has prepared for those who love Him! For now, you will need to be content with the Spirit's revealing only a sketchy framework of the big and broad picture of God's eternal plans. Bear in mind what His Word states regarding our limited ability to grasp His deeper thoughts and higher purposes for us. Accordingly we read: "For now we see in a mirror, dimly, but then face to face. Now I know in part, but then I shall know just as I also am known" (1 Corinthians 13:12).

Perhaps after your arrival at the *place* Jesus has prepared for you, there will be a "briefing" on your heavenly assignments. And then, progressively, the broad picture will unfold as, in joyful obedience, you begin to work out and walk out God's perfect destiny, to the praise of His glorious Name!

Prayer:

Thank You, Father God, and thank You, Lord Jesus, for the magnificent ministries of service You have prepared for me in Heaven. With joyful expectation, I will wait upon Your Holy Spirit to reveal them to me. I thank You for inspiring my spirit and giving me a vision filled with Your hopes and Your plans designed uniquely for me. In the Name of Jesus I pray. Amen.

HEAVEN IS A PLACE
WHERE GOD HIMSELF WILL
WIPE EVERY TEAR FROM
OUR EYES. HE HAS
PREPARED A PLACE FOR
YOU THERE, AND HE HAS
INVITED YOU TO COME.
BUT YOU HAVE TO RSVP!
HOW WILL YOU ANSWER
GOD'S INVITATION?

— **Anne Graham Lotz** —
From: *Heaven, My Father's House*, Inside cover

25

HOW TO SAY FINAL GOOD-BYES

Scripture:

Then Jacob saw Joseph's sons, and said, "Who are these?" And Joseph said to his father, "They are my sons, whom God has given me in this place." And he said, "Please bring them to me, and I will bless them." Now the eyes of Jacob were dim with age, so that he could not see. Then Joseph brought them near to him, and he kissed them and embraced them.

Genesis 48:8-10

Now this is the blessing with which Moses the man of God blessed the children of Israel before his death.

Deuteronomy 33:1

Meditation:

Can you surmise why the Holy Spirit, the author of the entire Bible, chose to include this story of Jacob blessing his grandsons with kisses and embraces? Or why are we permitted to eavesdrop on the tender and holy moments of Jacob and Moses as they spoke their final good-byes to their own children, as well as to the extended families of the children of Israel represented by the twelve tribes? I believe God's abiding intention through these stories is to provide for all succeeding generations, including our own, wise instruction and godly examples of how to speak final good-byes to our precious family. In doing so, you will learn how important it is to cement the bonds of love with those persons you treasure the most. The result will be a peaceful assurance that these relationships will endure for all time, transcend your earthly habitation, and extend eternally into the Kingdom of Heaven.

Frequently, medical professionals responsible for

the care of dying persons will notify the immediate family that their loved one has little time remaining. Such notices might include words similar to these: "If you want to pay a final visit at the bedside of your loved one, you need to make your way there now." My counsel to the person *for whom death is drawing near* is not to wait until your last days or last hours to ask your spouse, sons, daughters, and grandchildren (such as you have), to come to your room. Hopefully, they will respond *before* you become too weak to speak and to reach out your arms for a hug and a kiss. Remember the request Jacob spoke to his son Joseph: "Please bring [my two grandsons] and I will bless them."

What a tender, unforgettable moment it was for Joseph and those grandkids! To do the same for your nearest and dearest loved ones is a powerful way to bid them a memorable farewell. While you are still able, it is also important to communicate your love verbally. It is preferable to do so individually to each member of your family. Use spoken words, as best you can, to express the thoughts and emotions of your heart. Speak words that convey your blessings, as well as God's blessing. As graciously as possible, extend your good will and wishes for health, peace and prosperity to attend their future. There is power in the spoken word of blessings! The power of your love, coupled with the power of God's love, will be etched upon the heart, mind, and memory of each family member you bless. Release, and openly express your deep sorrow and grief. Freely pour out your heart and let the tears flow! That's what Jacob and Moses did! The Holy Spirit will give you the heart, the courage, the words and the strength to speak a holy good-bye that will keep on speaking long after you have parted from your earthly family and departed for God's family in Heaven above.

In southern Missouri, there is a wayside chapel just off U.S. Route 71. It's called the *Precious Moments Chapel.* Your Father God wants the room containing your bedside, in whatever setting, to become a "Precious Moments Chapel" where His Holy Presence will envelope you and your loved ones. The moments you and your family spend together privately expressing your mutual love, gratitude, and appreciation, verbally and nonverbally, will be most precious. They will be precious to you, your family, and to God Himself.

Prayer:

My Father, my God, Thank You for the wise

examples of Jacob and Moses, which have modeled for me how to say good-bye to my precious family. By Your Spirit, move upon me and free me to express with emotion and words from the depths of my heart the love and the gratitude that will seal the bond between us forever. Thank You for establishing the bonds of Your everlasting love into my heart through Jesus Christ. In His name I pray. Amen.

BUT EVEN WHEN
PEOPLE ARE TOO WEAK
TO SPEAK, OR HAVE LOST
CONSCIOUSNESS,
THEY CAN HEAR;
HEARING IS THE LAST
SENSE TO FADE

— **Maggie Callahan & Patricia Kelley** —
From: *Final Gifts*, pg. 50

26

RELEASING YOUR LOVED ONES

Scripture:

For He looked down from the height of His sanctuary; from Heaven the Lord viewed the earth, to hear the groaning of the prisoner, to release those appointed to death.

Psalm 102:19-20

Meditation:

How hard it is for each of you to stand by and observe the increasing intensity of your loved one's suffering. The reality of your impending loss has set in with increasing sorrow and grief. Imagine, if you can, how much harder it will be for your precious loved one to speak fondly, tenderly, and tearfully a final good-bye to each you. You are losing one person, while he or she is losing all of you! Quite possibly, the closing weeks and days will be accompanied by excruciating pain in the body causing a groaning in the soul and spirit as well. Perhaps you are being stretched in your own spirit beyond sympathy and empathy to the point of grasping for a way to absorb at least a portion of your loved one's anguish. There is a way of doing this.

Begin by taking heart! Hear again the Word of the Lord who: "From Heaven the Lord viewed the earth, to hear the groaning of the prisoner, to release those appointed to death" (Psalm 102:19-20). Yes! It is true. The Lord is hearing the groans of your loved one and has the power to *release* him or her from the prison of torturous pain and from the grip of death itself. Learning this truth, I trust that there is in your spirit a sigh of relief ready to be expressed with the words, "Thank God."

Not only is it necessary for the Lord to release those appointed to death, members of the family need to do the same! Here are some critically important and specific ways for you to express parting words to your dying loved one. I don't presume to put words in your mouth; I only offer to impress some *concepts* upon your mind. It is understandably true that the deeper, the stronger, and the longer is the bond you have shared with your loved one, the harder it will be for you to accept his or her death and endure the separation which immediately follows.

Consider these choice words used by Jesus to minister to the grief of separation His disciples were experiencing after He announced His departure to return to His Father in Heaven. "Therefore you now have sorrow; but I will see you again and your heart will rejoice, and your joy no one will take from you" (John 16:22). As Christians trusting in Jesus to come back and "see you again," your separation from your loved one, and your loved one from you, is *temporary*—temporary because God's love for His dear children is *powerfully permanent*! The love God has poured into your hearts for your loved one about to depart to be with his or her Father in Heaven is fully capable of enduring this temporary separation!

My reason for dwelling on God's enduring love is to prepare you to do a very hard thing: your need to *release* your precious loved one into God's everlasting arms. His arms are extended and waiting to embrace and welcome His beloved son or daughter to his or her eternal home in Heaven prepared by Jesus!

Through my many years of pastoral experience caring for the dying, together with their families, I have learned that some individuals really struggle to accept the impending death. This is particularly true when it occurs abruptly and/or prematurely. The result is a type of denial, which actually prevents them from releasing their precious one. Indeed, there are occasions when more than one member of the immediate family needs practical help to resist denial, accept the inevitable, and seal it by speaking words of release. Clinical studies have shown, in some cases, that the inability and failure to release a loved one can actually prolong the dying process. Those facing death have the need to hear from each member of the family that they are released to depart from their midst to be with the Lord.

In some circumstances, I have found it necessary, as a pastor, to lovingly exhort family members to speak (even to those in a comatose state), sincere and simple words of release and commendation. Such an expression can be very simple, such as: "I release you to go now and be with the Lord." In some instances when my counsel was heeded, a quiet and peaceful departure took place within a few days.

Releasing a loved one is not an easy task for a spouse and for sons and daughters. God is your Helper in the person of the Holy Spirit. Don't worry about saying the "right words." They may sound awkward, halting, and possibly be interrupted with sobs of uncontrollable weeping. This is more than okay; it is good—good for you and good for your loved one.

One concluding thought: your loved one, drawing nearer to the time of departure, has likely already read this meditation. If, after a time of your reading this meditation, you have not yet spoken your personal words of release, that loved one could very well be expecting you to do so. Please don't disappoint him or her!

Prayer:

Merciful God, by the example of Your Son Jesus, and by words of this meditation, You have prompted me to speak words of release and commendation to my dear loved one. I humbly admit that I cannot do this without Your help and strength. Thank You for the comfort of knowing that You will speak the final decree of release for my loved one, freeing this precious person from the prison of pain, grief, and death itself. In Your mercy, hear my cry. In the Name of Jesus I pray. Amen.

27

CHURCH BELLS MAY BE TOLLING NOW, BUT ONE DAY THEY WILL BE RINGING

Scripture:

Then Moses and the children of Israel sang this song to the Lord, and spoke, saying: 'I will sing to the Lord, for He has triumphed gloriously, the horse and its rider He has thrown into the sea! The Lord is my strength and song, and he has become my salvation; He is my God, and I will praise Him; my father's God, and I will exalt Him. Your right hand, O Lord, has become glorious in power; Your right hand, O Lord, has dashed the enemy in pieces.'

Exodus 15:1-2, 6

Concluding Meditation:

Four centuries is a long time for any ethnic group to be born to live and to die in slavery. Such was the fate of God's chosen people—the Hebrews who served under the oppressive hand of the kings of Egypt. "And the Lord said: 'I have surely seen the oppression of My people who are in Egypt, and have heard their cry because of their taskmasters, for *I know their sorrows*" (Exodus 3:7). [Emphasis added] Notice God's threefold response to His people's suffering. He responded with His *eyes*, His *ears*, and His *heart*. In the exact same manner, He is responding to the heavy taskmasters of disease, infirmities, injuries, disabilities, and the cruelest of them all, death that has afflicted His people of all ages. Be assured that God *sees* your oppression, *hears* your cries, and *knows* your sorrows!

Moses was God's great emancipator, bringing deliverance to many generations of enslaved

Hebrews. After four hundred years of tyrannical oppression, the day of deliverance for God's people finally dawned. Before that day's end, this multitude gathered at the Red Sea shore, gloriously amazed and jubilant, as they sang spontaneously a new song of praise to God for His gift of freedom!

Jesus is God's great Emancipator bringing deliverance from bondage to sin, sickness, and death. As a result of your particular disease, or perhaps a fatal injury, your body is held captive to pain, disablement, and eventually, death itself. In like manner, dear friend, the day of your deliverance is about to dawn! The oppressive days of cries and sighs, groaning and moaning, pains and strains will cease. Soon the host of saints and angels, numbering untold millions of millions standing at Heaven's shores will be singing joyously as they welcome you *HOME!* Your very first response might well be like unto the much-celebrated acclamation of Martin Luther King, Jr., who concluded his famous "I Have a Dream" speech by shouting with resounding glee: "Free at last! Free at last! Thank God Almighty, I'm free at last!" Listen with your spirit's ear. Can you hear them singing, though so very distant, yet so mystically near?

During more than a decade of missionary journeys to many nations on several continents, I considered it to be no small part of my mission to go prayer walking in cities, towns, and villages. One bright and beautiful fall day in the city of Panevezys, Lithuania, I came upon a large Catholic church. A funeral coach and hearse were parked at the end of a block-long brick walkway leading from the front entrance of the sanctuary to the courtyard exit. The funeral service had all but concluded as preparations were being made to begin the procession to the burial site.

I chose a place to watch and pray beneath a large spreading chestnut tree with leaves of pure gold glistening in the bright autumn sun. Soon numerous mourners emerged from the sanctuary and began to line the walkway on either side. Many of them were carrying large baskets of tribute flowers. Others came with a variety of potted plants, including lovely ferns and palms. The sight was impressive, dignified and beautiful. Presently, the brightly-vested clergy appeared, and were followed by the pallbearers escorting the casket, slowly and reverently walking down the magnificent walkway.

Suddenly, a huge bell in the towering church steeple began to toll. At first, the dominant, methodical *BONG-BONG-BONG,* which must have reverberated for a radius of several miles, generated within me feelings of heaviness, a sense of stark finality, and a veritable death knell. But soon this sound became to me a vivid realization of John Donne's famous words: "Never send to know for whom the bell tolls; it tolls for you." As this tolling continued, my feelings about the sound began to gradually change. The loud sound began to interpret for me tones of dignified somberness, followed by overtones of worshipful appropriateness, well-suited for the occasion.

Abruptly, the tolling was silenced. Immediately, an entirely new sound began to emanate from the same steeple tower. It filled the air, the ear, and the spirit. I soon recognized it to be the sound of a carillon! Not a single bell *tolling,* but many bells *ringing* melodiously and harmoniously a triumphant Easter hymn. Though I didn't know the words, inwardly my spirit was singing along with the carillon. It lifted me spiritually and caused me to look heavenward. A gentle breeze had begun to rustle the golden leaves of the chestnut trees in a waving motion. Then the Holy Spirit brought to my remembrance the words of the prophet Isaiah, who proclaimed: "For you shall go out with joy, and be led forth with peace; the mountains and the hills shall break forth into singing before you, and all the trees of the field shall clap their hands" (Isaiah 55:12).

Listen one more time to the "free-at-last" celebration song of the Hebrews at the Red Sea: "Your right hand, O Lord, has become glorious in power; Your right hand, O Lord, has dashed the enemy to pieces" (Exodus 15:6).

Yes, the enemy of death, which had been so fearsome to all of humanity for all the ages, has been dashed in pieces by the gloriously powerful right hand of the Lord Jesus Christ through His death and resurrection!

Dear friend, be sure to take this to heart, so that it may build your faith and fortify your courage. Jesus has indeed already broken the grab and the grip of your personal death! At God's appointed time for you to be released from your failing body, you likely will hear the bell *tolling* for you. But keep listening carefully with your inner ear of faith for the gladsome sounds of the carillon bells which will soon begin *ringing for you*! What song will they be singing? Perhaps this one: "For you shall go out with joy, and be led forth with peace; the mountains and the hills shall break forth into singing before you, and all the trees of the field shall clap their hands" (Isaiah 55:12).

Prayer

Precious Jesus, my Lord and my God: Thank You for Your powerful right hand which has gripped me and led me throughout my life, during the time of terminal illness, and now at the time of approaching death. Thank You for what You are about to do— leading me out of my pain, out of my sorrows and tears, triumphantly into Your promised land! Please comfort and bless my precious family of loved ones, and my faithful caregivers. Open our ears and tune our hearts to hear Your carillon bells ringing and singing a hymn of praise for Your saving grace. Yes, dear Jesus, with great expectation I long to *see* Your face and *feel* Your strong embrace! I pray this prayer in Your strong Name Jesus, You who are my resurrection and my life, even life eternal! Amen.

APPENDIX A

This is a ready reference of selected scriptures for administering pastoral care to those with the following needs:

Those who are sick and infirm
Those facing emergencies and uncertainties
Those enduring prolonged suffering
Those diagnosed with terminal illness

This resource identifies five appropriate scripture passages, which relevantly address each of the four types of needs for use by pastors, chaplains, hospice personnel, and other caregivers.

I – PASSAGES FROM GOD'S WORD FOR THE SICK AND INFIRM:

Isaiah 53:1-5 – Christ was crucified for sin *and sicknesses*

Psalm 103:1-3 – Forgiveness and healing in Christ is *total*

Psalm 34:15-19 – The righteous are also subject to afflictions

Matthew 14:13-21– The *compassion* of Jesus heals all

James 5:13-18 – The necessity of confessing sins to one another

II – PASSAGES FROM GOD'S WORD FOR THOSE FACING EMERGENCIES AND UNCERTAINTIES:

Psalm 46:1-11 – God's 911 emergency "hot line"

Matthew 14:22-33 – What to do when the storms roar

Luke 18:1-8 – God's "911" never connects to an answering machine

Philippians 4:4-9 – God's "prescription" for dealing with anxiety

I Peter 5:6-11 – Another "secret" for being released from anxiety

III – PASSAGES FROM GOD'S WORD FOR THOSE ENDURING PROLONGED SUFFERING:

Isaiah 40:28-31 – Man's extremity is God's opportunity

Romans 8:18-25 – What God *may* be saying through suffering

Mark 5:24-34 – The Great Physician does not deal in opinions

Romans 5:1-5 – Some of the *good* "side affects" of suffering

1 Peter 1:3-9 – Suffering *may* be God's way of building faith

IV – PASSAGES FROM GOD'S WORD TO COMFORT THE TERMINALLY ILL:

Psalm 23:1-3 – The Good Shepherd is always in full control

John 14:1-7 – Our eternal place with Jesus in Heaven

2 Corinthians 4:16-5:15 – Transition from "tent" to

"building"

Romans 8:31-39 – The inseparable bond of God's eternal love

Revelation 21:1-8 – All things are *being* made new

APPENDIX B

This is a ready reference of selected scriptures for ministering pastoral care to those with the following needs:

The Bereaved
The Lonely
The Depressed
The Weary

This guide is designed to provide five appropriate scripture passages which relevantly address each of the four types of needs to be used by pastors, chaplains, hospice personnel, and other caregivers as in **Appendix A.**

I – PASSAGES FROM GOD'S WORD FOR THE BEREAVED:

2 Samuel 12:15-23 – Comfort on the death of a child
Isaiah 40:1-8 – Comfort for the sorrowing
John 11:1-26 – Jesus is the Resurrection and eternal life
1 Thessalonians 4:13-18 – Grieving with hope
1 Corinthians 15:35-40 – The Resurrection of the body

II – PASSAGES FROM GOD'S WORD FOR THE LONELY. ESPECIALLY WIDOWS AND WIDOWERS:

Psalm 68:1-6 – God sets the lonely in families

Psalm 25:8-18 – The friendship of the Lord

Isaiah 41:8-10 – God stays close to His chosen people

Luke 7:11-16 – Widows have a special place in God's heart

James 1:27 – Pastors and elders have an important ministry to widows

III – PASSAGES FROM GOD'S WORD FOR THE DEPRESSED AND THE HOPELESS:

Psalm 42:1-11 - God's gift of hope for the hopeless

1 Thessalonians 5:16-24 – Being thankful in all circumstances

Isaiah 61:1-3 – The Holy Spirit mends broken hearts

1 Peter 1:3-9 – Believers are born anew to a living hope

1 Kings 19:9-18 – God seeks after the depressed and dejected

IV – PASSAGES FROM GOD'S WORD FOR THE WEAK AND WEARY:

Isaiah 40:28-31 – Learning to wait for the Lord

Isaiah 50:4-9 – The importance of ministering to the weary

Matthew 11:28-30 – Allowing Jesus to carry your burdens

Galatians 6:1-10 – The priority of rendering good deeds for believers

Hebrews 12:1-4 – Keeping our eyes on Jesus for more faith

About the Author

While serving as a member of the United States Army in Korea, God in His mercy, spared Glenn A. Pearson's life from fierce combat during the closing operations of the war. As an initial expression of gratitude, he committed his life to Christ Jesus and began to seek God's purpose for his life. During his second year of studies at the Lutheran Bible Institute in Minneapolis, Minnesota, he experienced a clear calling from God to prepare to serve Him as a pastor.

Upon completion of his under-graduate degree, he enrolled in the Lutheran School of Theology at the Rock Island, Illinois campus. In 1965, he received a master of divinity degree and was ordained into the Lutheran Church of America. For the next 30 years, Glenn enjoyed successful ministry as pastor of six churches in four states.

During the latter portion of this ministry, God began to open doors for him to serve as a missionary teacher training theological students, pastors, and church leaders in several nations abroad.

Upon retiring as a full-time parish pastor in 1995, Glenn began to make more frequent short-term missionary journeys abroad. To date, trips have been made to the following nations: India, Mexico, Nigeria, Kenya, Guatemala, Slovenia, Sweden, Estonia, Lithuania, Latvia, Belarus, Russia, and Pakistan.

To better facilitate this overseas mission, in 1997 Glenn founded a para-church ministry known as The Desire of All Nations Ministries, Inc. The purpose of this non-profit organization is to provide discipleship teaching and practical skills training for theological students, pastors and leaders of local churches. Additional ministries rendered include financial assistance and humanitarian aid in the form of medical supplies and equipment, nutritional supplements, and audio-visual equipment to facilitate evangelism programs.

Glenn and his wife Esther Ruth have been happily married for 45 years. God has blessed them with four daughters who are all believers in Christ with Christian husbands, and eleven grandchildren.

Printed in the United States
69800LV00003B/143-442